W9-CTA-760

AT
peace
WITH
PAIN

Dr. Claude M. Roberto & Dr. Paul S. Sussman

ENDORSED BY THE CHRONIC PAIN ASSOCIATION OF CANADA
EDMONTON 2006

PURCHASED AT UOFA MEDICAL BOOKSTORE NOV 6, 2007

© Copyright 2007 Roberto, Claude M.
Copyright on the drawings is held by the artists.

All rights reserved. No part of this publication may be used, produced, stored in a retrieval system, or transmitted in any forms or by any means, electronic, mechanical, photocopying, recording or otherwise, known and unknown, without the prior written permission of the copyright owners except in the case of brief quotations in critical articles and reviews.

First edition

Disclaimer: The authors do not endorse any one method of treatment and are not responsible for the outcomes of any therapies mentioned in this book. The authors, the Chronic Pain Association of Canada, the partners, colleagues, assistants, family, editors and publishers disclaim any liability in connection with use of this publication. They do not assume any responsibility or liabilities for any adverse effects, loss, injury, damage, illness, complications that may result from the practice of any activities or following any information or misuse of information or related information found in this book or on the websites and promotional material attached to this book. Readers are strongly advised to verify for themselves and investigate all items and information given in this book. Consult a physician before any of the actions or advice in this book are followed. Opinions presented in this book are the authors' opinions; some others are traditional. You, other people in pain, your physician and other health therapists might disagree with the information presented in this book.

This book was not sponsored by the pharmaceutical industry and the authors did not want the chapter on medications to be influenced by the ones producing the medications discussed in the book.

Address: Chronic Pain Association of Canada, Box 66017, Heritage Postal Outlet, Edmonton, Alberta, Canada T6J 6T4

Note for Librarians: A cataloguing record for this book is available from Library and Archives Canada at www.collectionscanada.ca/amicus/index-e.html
ISBN 1-4120-7073-2

Printed in Victoria, BC, Canada. Printed on paper with minimum 30% recycled fibre.
Trafford's print shop runs on "green energy" from solar, wind and other environmentally-friendly power sources.

TRAFFORD
PUBLISHING™

Offices in Canada, USA, Ireland and UK

Book sales for North America and international:
Trafford Publishing, 6E–2333 Government St.,
Victoria, BC V8T 4P4 CANADA
phone 250 383 6864 (toll-free 1 888 232 4444)
fax 250 383 6804; email to orders@trafford.com
Book sales in Europe:
Trafford Publishing (UK) Limited, 9 Park End Street, 2nd Floor
Oxford, UK OX1 1HH UNITED KINGDOM
phone 44 (0)1865 722 113 (local rate 0845 230 9601)
facsimile 44 (0)1865 722 868; info.uk@trafford.com
Order online at:
trafford.com/05-1984

10 9 8 7 6 5 4 3 2

Note to the reader:

This book is based on personal experiences. Therapies found in this book may not give you the same results we experienced.

The book is meant to help inform readers about various techniques in the field of pain therapy. The authors are not physicians. Dr. Roberto's starting point for this publication was her personal experience with chronic pain caused by a car accident in 1997. Dr. Roberto wrote the book and later she invited Dr. Sussman to join her writing project because of his experience with chronic pain caused by a car accident in 1971. In addition, Dr. Roberto is Francophone and she needed assistance from Dr. Sussman to offer quality control to her English manuscript. Of course the book is not meant to substitute for professional face-to-face advice; each individual is unique. One always does well to inform one's doctors of any and all treatments one may be following. This assists you and your caregivers to develop and maintain a good pain management plan. You always do well to consult a physician before starting any therapy. The book does not necessarily reflect the ideas or thinking of other authors or health providers.

This book will encourage you to take an active role, to look at your pain from different angles. It will give you the tools you may use to improve quality of life. It will allow you to reach goals set in your healing plan and to include the essential in your therapy; it strives to help you find a meaning in your pain. The techniques for finding well-ness are accessible to everybody and are meant to empow-er. Select the ones you prefer and discuss them with your team. The book is not written to be read from beginning to the end, but rather to be opened wherever you want. Please consult it when needed and use the index in order to find your way in the complexity of pain. We want you to feel better and we do not defend one therapy more than anoth-er; we invite you to make informed decisions on which methods you include in your quest for good health. You are in charge of your life and well-being.

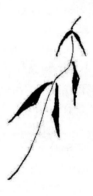

To all the ones experiencing pain.

To tell them love is stronger than pain,
otherwise there would be no book.

Claude M. Roberto was born in Southern France. She now lives in Edmonton in Western Canada. She had an academic teaching and research career in Humanities at the University of Ottawa and also at the University of Alberta where she received a Ph.D. in Classical Archaeology in 1984. She became an advocate in healing from pain after having a serious car accident in 1997 in front of a local playground for children. After this accident, she placed healing as a top priority, an action that has changed her life for ever. She is now Vice-President of the Chronic Pain Association of Canada, a national organization aiming at improving chronic pain treatment and facilitating the lives of hundreds of thousands of Canadian and North American people living with pain. She offers workshops and presentations to persons in pain, medical and pharmaceutical students as well as physicians wishing to upgrade their knowledge of treating chronic pain. She teaches pain recovery strategies and gives hope to those who contact the Chronic Pain Association of Canada for assistance. She also meets with decision makers and politicians to improve legislation so that clients and physicians have more power in treating pain. In addition, she is often involved with clinical trials aimed at finding new and improved medication for the ones in pain. This book contains information gathered from these various experiences and from her personal life as someone experiencing constant chronic pain. Claude is known to tell her readers or public how to enjoy life even if it is full of pain; she never tells them how to get totally rid of it because pain can be intractable. However she explains how to reduce pain with different techniques and how to avoid to see preoccupation for pain being a focus in life because healing is then impossible. In spite of her busy life as well as the intractable pain caused by her head and spinal injuries, Claude is always willing to travel and improve the life of people in pain. She received several academic awards and literary prizes for previous books as well as in 2004 a Queen Elizabeth II's Golden Jubilee Award given to outstanding Canadians for inspiring others, improving their life conditions and volunteering for communities at the local and national levels.

Paul S. Sussman was born in Berkeley, California and now lives in Edmonton, Alberta, Canada. He was awarded a B.A. in Psychology at California State University at San Jose, and the M.A. and Ph.D. in Psychology at Carleton University in Ottawa, Canada. Paul is the founder and creative force behind Sussman Psychological, one of the oldest established psychology clinics in Alberta. Paul is licensed in Alberta and the State of Georgia. He specializes in treating chronic conditions such as pain and addiction, post-traumatic adjustment, and the so-called personality disorders. Paul is not a medical modeler; rather he adheres to an alternative pattern based upon principles of growth and development. He wants to improve the quality of life of his clients in pain and facilitate their access to adequate resources. He emphasizes expression of feelings, also called emotional release; he views wellness as most readily achieved not through treatment and cure, but through human connection, interaction, and becoming. He uses breathing to bring an altered state of consciousness allowing recovery of past inner issues increasing chronic pain and preventing healing; when these past experiences come back to his clients, Paul is able to discover the meaning of their pain and to suggest ways to dissolve these issues and decrease pain. He believes pain is a tool to understand and solve deeply buried issues. Healing is then not a treatment but it is a transformation because it positively impacts the physical body as well as emotions. Paul has a long experience in music and broadcasting radio programs; he has authored a very large number of important scientific and lay publications in North America, and he holds numerous awards, including the Presidents' Award from the Psychologists' Association of Alberta, for his significant contributions to Psychology.

He is a member of the Chronic Pain Association of Canada endorsing this publication.

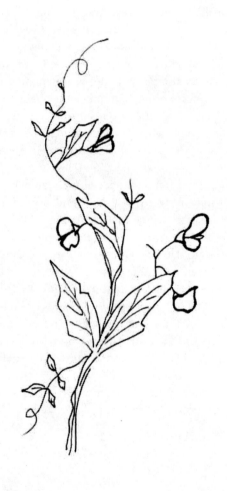

CONTENTS

Acknowledgments

Claude wishes to thank many friends, doctors and therapists who cared for her and contributed to the writing of this book. These caregivers and teachers include Dr. Barbara Wood, Dr. Janet Chiu, Dr. Darrell Smith, Dr. Michele Sawatzky, Dr. Roger Gervais, Margaret Penner-Poncilius, Christy Kasur, Cynthia Christenson, Brent Morrow, Marcel Dusyk, Tamara Bliss, Miriam Esquitin and Wendy Gervais. Paul wishes to thank his many clients, friends and therapists for providing inspiration. Claude and Paul put into the book their own practical experiences from being injured in two different car accidents (none was their fault) and they are grateful to their lawyers, Robert Simpson, Debbie Miller and Len Pollock who unconditionally supported them in the legal system. They added to this publication the experience of others contacting them for pain relief, all the teachings received from numerous therapists, in addition to a more academic knowledge of pain based on scientific research projects.

Thanks also go to Dr. Pierre Flor-Henry, Clinical Director at the Alberta Hospital Edmonton, who read the manuscript and offered positive comments encouraging the authors to turn their writings into a publication; Dr. Helen Hays, Associate Clinical Professor at the University of Alberta in Edmonton and an exceptional world class pain specialist who developed palliative care in Western

Canada, for her Preface, committed support and ongoing care; Barry Ulmer, our tireless and dedicated Executive Director at the Chronic Pain Association of Canada, for writing the Foreword; Heather Divine, President of the Chronic Pain Association of Canada, Dianne Tomm-Lunty and the late Catherine Ireland, Directors of this same Association, and friends as well as survivors from the Chronic Pain Association of Canada for sharing their stories and for their ongoing encouragement and inspiration. These therapists and friends were the first ones to read and bring constructive criticism to the project. They deserve unlimited thanks for their trust and support.

A special thank you goes to Amélie Roberto-Charron, a 16 year-old talented and fabulous teenager, and to Ariane Roberto-Charron, a 13 year-old brilliant girl, for being sources of inspiration; another thank you goes to Dr. Eugène Roberto for drawing most illustrations found in the book; and to the staff at Trafford Publishing for their professionalism in turning the manuscript into a successful book.

Claude Roberto, Ph.D.
Paul Sussman, Ph.D.

Preface

Dr. Claude M. Roberto is a great inspiration to others and indeed to the medical profession who can learn from her experience.

Chronic pain whether due to a malignancy and a life threatening condition, or due to a chronic condition caused by accident, congenital disability or other systemic illness is a hidden plague of our times. Some recent surveys have found that up to at least 20% of the Canadian population suffer chronic pain. Chronic neuropathic pain is becoming recognized as an illness in its own right.

Chronic noncancer pain (CNCP) almost always has a strong component of central or peripheral nervous system damage. The damage is not always identifiable by sophisticated technology such as MRIs, CT scans, ultrasound, nerve conduction studies and so on. This being so, the pain may be discounted by the insurance industry, some professionals, and the general public.

An example of this is so-called whiplash injury (flexion extension injury). The sufferer may recover in months if the injury is relatively minor, but more serious collisions continue to cause physical distress indefinitely.

The cause of the pain is due to damage or complete disruption of many small nerve fibers, crushed or fractured vertebrae, disrupted intervertebral discs. On occasion surgery is done urgently, but may not help to reduce the pain.

Medically, the best chance of preventing ongoing chronic neuropathic pain is to continue normal activity as much as possible. This helps as much as physical therapy.

Anticonvulsant medications such as gabapentin (Neurontin), pregabalin (Lyrica), and topiramate (Topamax) may be helpful. If warranted, the attending physician may try stronger analgesics in the same class as morphine, or a combination of the above two classes of drugs. All of these medications have side effects. Medications are unlikely to reduce pain be more than one-third.

The main aims of medications are to reduce the pain to a score of five out of ten or less on a visual analog scale, with 0 as "no pain" and "10" as the most severe pain imaginable, and to promote enough relief for a better sleep (chronic pain affects all aspects of the person's life).

This brief discussion leads me to the praise that Dr. Claude M. Roberto deserves for writing this eloquent self-help book. She describes how she was able to overcome much of her disability while continuing her caring role of mother and wife and to continue her day-time job.

Dr. Helen Hays, MD, CCFP, FCFP
Associate Professor, Department of Family Medicine,
University of Alberta
Canada

Foreword

The under treatment of pain in Canada has led us to refer to it as the "silent epidemic," which conveys the magnitude and overall lack of understanding of this debilitating, life altering disease.

Pain is common. A large portion of the Canadian population suffers from pain and pain is the most common reason individuals seek health care. Each year, an estimated 5 million Canadians suffer chronic pain and another 2.5 million experience acute pain due to injury or surgery. Chronic pain is the most common cause of long-term disability, and almost one third of all Canadians will experience chronic pain in their lives. As we age the number of us who will require treatment for pain from back disorders, degenerative joint diseases, rheumatologic conditions, and a multitude of other reasons, will increase. Yet, there is ample evidence that pain continues to be mistreated, misunderstood, and often maligned as not being real.

When I first became involved in the "pain field" there was very little information available to those suffering. Few doctors would even see you on a continuing basis, and fewer still had any knowledge about pain. Most pain sufferers were called malingerers, some referred to as "drug seekers" and almost all ended up in the doctor shuffle. Has the situation changed today?

Some will tell you yes, others will tell you a little bit, yet others are still caught in the doctor shuffle, not receiving any help at all.

What has changed is the growing body of evidence that pain is under treated and the volume of information that is now available; but the perspective from a pain patient point of view is still in short supply.

This book, *At Peace with Pain*, will be a major boon for those who suffer and it fills in many of the numerous blanks that surround the management of this debilitating disease. It outlines the journey of a pain patient through this most difficult condition and gives, not only hope, but many ideas and methods we can follow to help cope with pain.

I am very grateful to Dr. Claude M. Roberto and Dr. Paul S. Sussman for taking the time to give us all this account of her journey and an insight into the what we can all do to cope with and manage our pain.

Anyone who reads this ground breaking book will come away feeling much less helpless and definitely with more hope there is a "light" at the end of the tunnel.

Barry D. Ulmer
Executive Director
Chronic Pain Association of Canada
Box 66017, Heritage Postal Outlet, Edmonton, Alberta, Canada T6J 6T4

INTRODUCTION

> **Work against pain, and you lose.**
> **Work with pain, and the struggle**
> **lightens. The body is not the enemy.**
>
> Jackson, 2003, p. 357.

A Christmas celebration in Edmonton, Alberta, Canada. A warm home protected by two blue spruces, sprinkled with snow, and dressed for the holiday season with a wreath on the door, the traditional cheerful poinsettias on the piano and evergreen branches decorating a crystal chandelier that seems to call you inside. Imagine hordes of children, wearing new party clothes, passing in front of the Christmas tree loaded with lights and presents, laughing and running up and down the stairs. The smell of cinnamon and oranges takes over the front hallway, while the kitchen invites you with delicate scents of chocolate and nuts.

In the middle of festivities, I try to hold a conversation with my friend. I mention writing a book on chronic pain. I say the two words ... the conversations close to me seem to stop. Mentioning pain amid this happy gathering of good friends appears almost indecent. The children approach and fill their plates before sitting in front of the fireplace. I see my daughters sharing olives and shortbread, two of their favorite foods. Children don't care about pain now; after all tonight is Christmas. Tomorrow morning they will open shiny multicolored boxes under the tree. For them the past does not exist, today is wonderful and tomorrow will be even better.

Why a book on pain? Simply because pain and happiness are connected; each is an essential part of life. That living forces us to meet pain is one of the truths in the universe. Pain allows transformation. Making peace with pain ensures happiness. A book on chronic pain then is a book on happiness.

Again conversations compete with the laughter of children. I pay closer attention to the lights and the red wooden figures on the Christmas tree. Pain can be compared with all these decorations and even with the holiday spirit. Both pain and Christmas call up memories from past years and even past generations. These pile up and may overwhelm you.

Many homemade decorations are very old, like this straw angel with a harp, which could have belonged to grandparents who are not here tonight but still remembered. Other objects, more recent reminders of happy moments, could originate from time spent with a caregiver or in a daycare. Each one is unique. Even reminiscences of sad moments illuminate the tree.

Chronic pain is the same: over the years, when your body slowly degenerates, pain may gradually accumulate. Pain can overwhelm you with sad memories from your distant past before the illness, before the wounds. Ultimately one hurts not only because of recent illnesses but also because of other old injuries visiting again. When you are in pain, in the middle of the night, even old stories of suffering told by grandparents and other friends or relatives may come alive in your present. Of course the past holds pleasant memories too; happy moments are woven with painful ones… just like stories of miscarriages and successful pregnancies. However when pain strikes, old wounds tend to reopen and increase the intensity of our discomfort.

This book is meant to assist you if you struggle to decrease suffering and to heal. It considers the varied and complex therapies available for removing the suffering from pain. We do not want you to hurt any more. We hope your pain will decrease and you will become healthier because of the information you acquire. We wish also to share our personal experiences to give you strength and hope. We want the book to be your companion in your personal quest for peace and health.

Increasingly our society accepts different healing traditions. As a result, several medical systems and treatments are now available. Presenting a variety of options is important because people in pain often try different approaches before finding one that works. You try a treatment and observe results. If it is not helpful, you select another option. Sometimes a combination of two or three therapies is essential. How do you manage to try an option if you ignore most of what is available? Pain is a completely subjective phenomenon. While we wish to make our descriptions of responses to treatments accurate, these descriptions are as subjective as is pain. We will share with you our experiences with several therapies, but please keep in mind you may experience different responses from these same treatments. We avoid using the term "patient" and prefer the word "client" because we believe in an active role for anyone in pain.

No one wins anything from suffering and the book is not meant to make victims of us; one could argue that it is all karma. Even if we suspect pain is highly unfair, on the other hand the book is intended to make you feel hopeful and less lonely, maybe even better than before issues relating to pain entered your life.

We know that healing brings along peace with pain and it is hard to know if peace comes after or before healing. We believe they hold each other's hands and travel together. But how would you define healing and wellness? Where would you find it? How do you know if you are well when someone can be in a state of wellness while dying peacefully?

First of all, healing is at once both magical and ordinary. It can appear anywhere during any of your activities because hugs or a change in your life environment can heal you. It can rise from very little, it is connected to love and erases hopelessness.

Secondly please do not attempt to control something uncontrollable like pain because you might lose the fight and for sure this loss will increase your pain. You cannot open fire upon pain because it would be a form of suicide: how could you have a "battle with cancer" when this illness is so much a part of yourself? Or how could you declare a war to pain when it flows in your blood, creates lumps in your lymphatic system, jams your cells, irritates your bones, lives in your nerves and muscles, multiplies trigger points and muscle spasms in the deepest areas and when it is so intimate with your brain? It is impossible to throw away pain because starting as a parasite or a virus living in your body, it became part of your body, mind and spirit. Even if disease steals health, vitality and quality of life, when we look for healing, we should see pain more as a collaborator tuning us inward rather than as a thief.[1] A positive attitude can definitely mitigate pain, as long as you see the hope of benefit. In addition, how could you disconnect yourself from the flow of pain, coming from your far and recent past to make such an impact on your current life? If your illness is genetic, how could you consider your parents, your grandparents and other previous generations, at the origin of your pain, to be your enemies? If you look for peace in the family and harmony in your life, you cannot make opponents of your ancestors. We hope this book will direct your perception into new interpretations of pain as a sort of ally, or a traveling companion, perhaps not welcomed but accepted; an ally that we choose to tolerate in order to make peace and to heal.

We trust this book will guide you through the complexity of pain. Many circles are present in the world of pain where muscle spasms pull joints apart and where joints reply by causing more spasms. And what about getting up when feeling stiff, in order to decrease pain because of slow movement? What about being visited again by pain after a rest? Pain is capricious and has no boundary. It can be caused by numerous factors. However we can be sure of something: whatever the causes of pain, peace and healing are always possible; acceptance and gratitude are always options.

The first chapter describes pain and its many ramifications. The second chapter focuses on myths and facts relevant to pain. It also strives to improve your knowledge of pharmaceutical medications available on the market. The third chapter on physical therapies opens new doors on activities and health professionals to include in a recovery plan. The fourth chapter, on psychological care, examines the role of the mind and psychotherapies in pain management. The fifth chapter on energy medicine discusses untraditional therapies. It describes healing energies and explains approaches provided by alternative medicine; it explains the importance of the invisible and it serves as an introduction to energy medicine that is a new and growing field in the area of healing. The sixth chapter on connections concerns the need to develop a mission or purpose in life, and the importance of connecting with significant ones, communities, co-workers and medical teams. This chapter also illustrates how we are all a small part of the universe that must be shared if we wish to feel better. Our individual mission is an essential part of our life because it ensures permanent peace with pain. The conclusion will help you to define healing and happiness as well as to find them in your own life.[2]

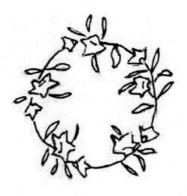

JULY 5, 2017

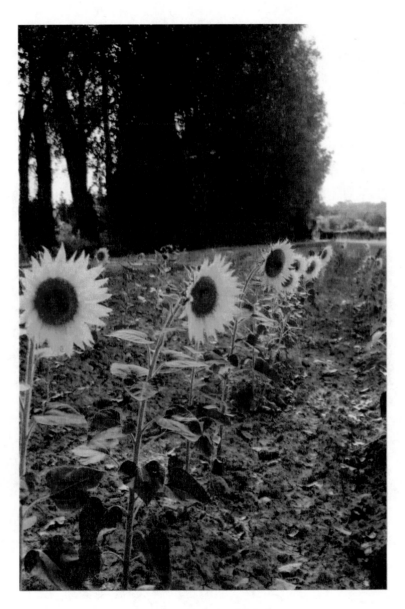

Orange, France, 2006.
Sunflowers know how to remain positive and always look for
the sun. Photo by Dr. Claude Roberto.

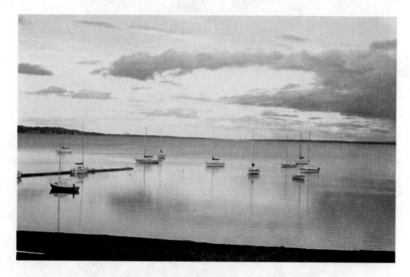

Away from pain. Calm coming back after a storm on
Wabamum Lake, Alberta, Canada, 2004.
Photo by Dr. Claude Roberto.

Chapter I

THE PAIN

HOW TO DESCRIBE PAIN

A challenge to define

> Pain is a more terrible Lord of mankind than even death.
>
> Albert Sweitzer

Pain is an invisible and personal condition that, perhaps because it does not leave one visibly disfigured, is often misunderstood. Although it is a universal human experience, pain remains extremely difficult to define. The experience of chronic pain is a long and scary journey quite often into the unknown: it hurts physically and mentally, it affects the body, the heart, the mind and the soul; it keeps invading life space. It costs money, steals quality of life, and destroys relationships. Pain is also a major expense and drain on economic and human resources. Traditional medical treatment places someone in pain in a passive role, waiting to consult a specialist, waiting for treatments to control symptoms, waiting for specific examinations, wait-

DEC. 5, 2007

ing for new scientific discoveries, waiting for hope, waiting for a cure, waiting for care, waiting for love, waiting for death...always waiting for everything. A person suffering in pain rarely smiles happily: moments of joy disappear quickly. New skills are needed to survive in a changing world. These must be practiced and mastered to remain functional in a society where self-sufficiency and independence are essential. Alone and lonely, we have one constant invisible companion: the pain, sometimes for an entire life.

> **Cries for help prove mostly useless. The person in pain belongs to a world that no one else can entirely share or comprehend.**
> Chronic Pain Association of Canada Newsletter, Volume 5, Issue 3, Fall 2001, p. 3.

Because happy painless moments fade and go away quickly even memories are affected. The very idea of a world without pain disappears; no one knows where or how, but it is gone, no longer conceivable. The one experiencing pain lives a mutilated existence and, if death does not come, one fights for a share of a dislocated existence in an unfriendly, unmanageable world. Life becomes a terrifying nightmare from which one may never truly awaken ... or a waking state in which the nightmare never ends.[1]

The complexity of pain

From a scientific perspective, pain proves difficult to quantify. Pain is a physical sensation, an emotional experience and a intruding response to a fear, injury or infection.[2] It can be consid-

> **Absence of evidence does not mean evidence of absence.**
> Jovey, 2002, p. VII.

ered to be the body's way to express emotions.[3] It affects the body, but also the soul, mind and emotions. For Plato pain was physical in addition to being an experience in the soul.[4] It can be called "a symphony" and considered "a complex dynamic involving not only pain sensors but emotions, memory and hormones."[5]

Pain can be sorted neatly into two main types, one of which may be further divided into two subcategories. The first type is pain that carries no new information. This is chronic pain, like the lower back pain some people experience even early on in life. One does well to get medical help, and to learn to tune this kind of pain out. This book will give you ideas to reduce this pain. It is not helpful to focus on it; in fact, focusing on chronic pain risks creating an obsessive preoccupation. Anyone, young or old, may have chronic pain. If it becomes a neurotic preoccupation, you have trouble indeed.

The second type is pain that signals new information; usually that you are being injured right now. This type of acute pain is divided into two basic subcategories: one, such as burning the hand on the stove, is accidental; the other, such as extracting a tooth, is a result of planned action. The first subcategory indicates an immediate danger, the second one shows we are approaching a goal we have in mind.

Pain is rarely caused by just one factor. Physical and psychological manifestations of pain are interlocked, our bodies can hurt our spirits and souls, and vice-versa.[6] There are at least two components of pain, the physiological component found in the neurological pathways, and the suffering (emotional and psychological) component that often is the hardest to bear and treat.[7] Suffering takes place when emotions are out of control and when tasks are impossible

to perform. Sometimes only the first component is treated and the second one is often forgotten. In a good pain
management program both, physical issues and suffering,
must be addressed. Both can be reduced with different
therapies which the client should try one after the other
or in a combined program. Alternative medicine is good
because it can heal and reduce suffering even if it cannot
remove all physical pain. However, the painkillers that are
America's preferred method of pain relief,[8] are also essential in most cases and help alternative medicine to give
better results. Chronic pain rarely disappears, it usually
decreases or comes back as flare-ups. The essential task in
the treatment of chronic pain is to render life more enjoyable through reducing the pain level without causing too
many side effects.

Pain is also considered, in medical terms, to be "a dis-
sociative experience" causing us to be separated from what
is surrounding us.[9] In other words, pain changes your relationship with the world. All pain is real, it is not "in the
head" such as commonly mentioned when no damage
to body tissues can be demonstrated. We can say it is the
product of the brain or the result, in some cases, of emotional issues. Nevertheless, even if no one can legitimize
your suffering with a number or a scan or a picture, pain
is very rarely faked.[10]

Subjective by definition, pain can only be known by the
person experiencing it. Measurement is generally on the
basis of personal report. Many factors influence the perception of pain, including lifestyle, mood, temperament,
mechanisms of the body sustaining the pain, meaning
of pain and psychological factors, such as a person's coping skills, responses to pain acceptable in the family and
cultural group, previous pain experiences and emotional

support. Sensations vary with stress and while most people share about the same pain threshold, pain tolerance varies hugely according to each person's beliefs, emotional responses and the surrounding circumstances.[11] This means that one person can have a different pain threshold and tolerance under different circumstances. There is no specific organ attached to pain such as ear or eye. Pain is an individual interpretation of sensory experience. With respect to gaining an empirically based understanding of pain, there is no specific sense organ to study.

The emotional side of pain

All disquieting emotions can be sorted in a similar fashion to physical pain. There are seven primary emotions, six of them disquieting: glad, mad, sad, afraid, ashamed, hurt, lonely. All disquieting emotions have the nothing new form; the right now but I volunteered for this form; and the get me out of here or get that away from me form. For example sad: There is the kind of sad that you are because a parent died; the kind of sad you are right at the time your parent was dying; and the kind of sad you are while you break up with someone because it has to be done.

> No two pains are the same, no two people experiencing pain have the same experience. It is very, very personal and individual.
>
> Dr. Helen Hays, pain specialist.

Chronic pain always stirs up emotions. Even when we are happy and laugh, tears come to the eyes and indicate pain is always present, even if hidden inside ourselves. The word "pain" comes from a Latin word meaning "punishment." There is no punishment without emotions.[12] In 1946 Lieutenant Colonel Henry Beecher, a pioneer in placebo research and an anesthesiologist in the army during World War II, interviewed very seriously wounded soldiers. Several of them did not feel any pain. Beecher concluded that a soldier's wound releases him from war and lets him believe his troubles are over whereas with a civilian's accident it is the beginning of a disaster. Beecher was one of the first modern scientists to suggest that emotional feelings have an impact on experience of physical injury.[13] Feelings of hopelessness, rejection, anger and anxiety are commonly associated with chronic physical pain. These feelings lead to depression that can masquerade as a change in appetite, lack of energy, insomnia or restlessness or guilt. Depression is always a threat to a person with chronic pain especially if there is little or no family or social support in place. Depression can magnify pain and pain can intensify depression. The two feed each other and potentially create a dangerous vicious circle.[14] Any strategy for controlling pain that focuses upon the physical domain to the exclusion of the emotional, mental and spiritual domain risks more than being ineffectual. Taking a purely pharmacological approach to pain can well become dangerous because it does not solve hidden issues.

Disconnection between clients and doctors

Physicians are trained to cure illnesses and may find it difficult to treat people, especially when they believe there is no cure. It is also difficult to work as a team with other physicians on complex conditions. Clients (on the other

> When he takes me in his arms, he tells me loving words and I see life through pink glasses.
>
> Edith Piaf, French singer who experienced chronic pain.

hand) want to receive care. They want to choose life. They do not want to be a file. They want to be heard and touched. They want hope. It is unfortunately the case that many doctors, especially the ones who did not hear the word pain too often in medical school and/or have had little personal experience with pain, are trained for the illness, not for the person. They see the disease and are not trained to deal with or even to see the entire person. So a gap, too often immense and very dark, is created between the consumer and the medical system. This is apt to cause feelings of anger and depression, amplifying the pain. Of course there are exceptions with physicians seeing the entire person, however our traditional medical schools do not train medical students to connect with people in pain.

TIME AND PAIN

Our bodies are not made for chronic pain. The human experience of pain is distinct from that of other animals. One major reason for this seems to lie in the human capacity to bind time. Only human beings think in terms of yesterday and tomorrow.

Among the creatures of the earth, the human capacity to bind time is evidently unique. Only people do it. Even if it is argued that animals have this capacity, it clearly is not the case that they have it to the degree that people do. Only people keep a written history. Of all the creatures of the earth,

> It's not the pain of the past that stings me most, But the suffering the future holds; for men's minds, Once they have bred evil, breed only evil.
>
> Sophocles, Greek play writer, *Philoctetes*, 496 - 406 B.C.

humankind is the only one for whom their own existence is a problem, a mystery. It can be argued that people are the only beings on this planet for whom finding meaning in their lives is imperative. Perhaps animals do this as well; however they do not do it in the same manner as people do ... Not at all. Unfortunately this selfsame specifically human mental capacity to think in terms of history (past, present and future), this selfsame human need to find meaning in the mystery of their own existence can and does easily interact with any lasting experience of pain, increasing the difficulty of coming to terms with it.

Another factor differentiating the human experience of pain from the animal experience of pain may be found in the fact that people seek meaning in events. Perhaps animals do this as well; however they do not do it in the same manner as people do.

Whatever animals experience, they experience in the now. If there is a thorn in their foot now or a porcupine quill in their face now, they attend to it ... not in the way that people do, with their focus on the possible meanings and implications of the discomfort. But, they attend to it. However, if the thorn or the quill is not there now, they do not attend to it at all. It is unlikely that animals could experience chronic pain in the same emotional way that people do. Contrast this to the human condition.

For people, especially adults, living in the now is a challenge. Although we can only act in the present, we find it very difficult to live in the present; our minds and our attention are usually upon the past or the

> It (pain) has no future but itself,
> Its infinite realms contain Its
> past, enlightened to perceive New
> periods of pain.
>
> Emily Dickinson, poet who lived with
> chronic pain, 1830 - 1886.

future. We spend most of our time reflecting upon the meaning of events in the past, and anticipating events in the future. We feel guilt, remorse, anger and happiness about our memories. We feel anxiety and excitement about the future. Feelings emerging from our ideas about "not-now" comprise the vast majority of what we feel at any given "now." For humans, a thorn in the foot or a quill in the face does more than hurt right now. Feelings of regret and shame (about having been stupid or clumsy or mind-less enough to get injured in the first place) combine with feelings of anxiety (about possible scarring, incapacity, infection, and horrendous possible outcomes to injury including chronic ones) in a way that magnifies our expe-rience beyond the pale of anything another animal might have. Of course, our constructions concerning past and future events are always with us. Pain emerging from these constructions is chronic by definition.

> The future is darkness. No human mind can know it. It is best to live in the moment, live for today.
>
> From Jocasta to Oedipus, Sophocles, *Oedipus the King*, 1235 – 1236.

The mental capacity to bind time and to seek meaning in events emerges in the context of a biological system that is not designed to deal with anything chronic. For example, the system that mediates the biological response to stress (technically referred to as the hypothalamic pituitary-adre-nocortical axis) is particularly well suited for dealing with acute stressors with responses such as fighting and fleeing. Unfortunately, such responses are poorly suited to chronic causes and conditions. As a result, we human beings are physically vulnerable to the down side of our remarkable intellectual abilities. Compared with other species, human discomfort is more likely to become chronic; yet our bodies deal poorly with chronic discomfort.

CBC " Q " WRINSTON CHURCH rur RArTos
11:00 TO 11:33

NO PAINLESS HEALING

Three hundred year-old western medical philosophy supports the ideas that healing is painless because of technical improvement; chronic pain is useless; the ones experiencing chronic pain do not achieve anything. In addition, clients and physicians hope for a day when specialized techniques result in instant, painless healings like "Bones" McCoy can do on Star Trek. Unfortunately comfort is fragile and life is not so easy for people in pain: the recovery curve for factual and real healing is long, time consuming, and goes up on a gentle, wavy slope; it requires hard work and conditions such as the right environment and the right connections to help the ones in pain to feel better. Recovery does not depend solely on technology and medication even if a mythic vertical line is marketed by those who follow a "scientific" approach. A vertical healing line, without any physical and mental work, puts the client in a failing position. Healing takes place but progress is never vertical. The real growth curve goes up slowly and is never the same for everybody. This book will help you to climb on the right and gentle slope.

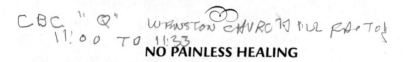

The two recovery curves: _____ indicates
the real curve we recommend in this book _ _ _ _ _ _ _ _

indicates the mythic curve

THE CAUSES OF OUR PAIN

Pain is caused by a myriad of reasons and conditions. It can be described with various degrees from 1 to 10 (ten being the highest level) and different adjectives, but pain can be felt only by the person suffering from it. Terms most often used to describe pain include the following words: flickering, quivering, beating, jumping, flashing, pricking, boring, drilling, cutting, lacerating, mild, discomforting, aching, constant, intermittent, deep, superficial, intense, dull, tugging, wrenching, hot, scalding, tingling, smarting, stinging, hurting, heavy, taut, rasping, splitting, tiring, exhausting, sickening, suffocating, fearful, frightful, terrifying, punishing, grueling, cruel, vicious, killing, wretched, binding, annoying, troublesome, miserable, intense, unbearable, spreading, penetrating, piercing, tight, numb, drawing, squeezing, tearing, cool, cold, freezing, nagging, nauseating, agonizing, dreadful, torturing, sharp, electrical, lightening bolts, pressing, sore, pounding, cramping, tight, crushing, piercing, knot-like, pinching, pins and needles, pulling, shooting, stretching, tender, trigger points, gnawing, swollen, stinging, distressing, horrible, excruciating, burning, stabbing, lancinating, searing, radiating, pulsing, throbbing, prickly, itchy, waves of pain, and many other words exist. Sometimes pain is perceived on the inside of the body. It can move from one place to another, it can appear and disappear for no reason at any time of the day or the night; it can surprise you with new ways to feel it; it can hurt the most on a particular place and hurt less on the rest of the body. It can be also permanent. In the simplest case pain comes from something that is dangerous such as heat from a stove or cut from a knife.[15]

Pain can be connected to arthritis, rheumatoid illness, lupus, fibromyalgia, trauma, car accident, injury to a nerve or any other short tissue, several types of neuromuscular disorders and syndromes, carpal tunnel, interstitial cystitis, colitis, cancer, scoliosis, burns, stones, loss of balance, migraine and headaches, endometriosis and premenstrual syndrome, psychological issues, stress increasing muscle tension and causing pain; it can be linked to a specific disease or disorder, or to treatments or to an injury. It is also influenced by how we feel emotionally.

> Then, the first wave of pain. He gasped. It was as if a hatchet lay lodged in his leg, slicing through each nerve with a hot blade. In his agony he perceived the word "fire" and felt flames licking at the torn bone and flesh. He tried to move, and could not. The pain grew.
>
> Lowry, 1993, p. 109.

In some cases pain arises from no reason. The brain manages the pain experience and allows the pain to be felt or to disappear according to distractions, emotions and other experiences. Therefore it is normal for pain to vary in intensity. Modern sophisticated equipment allows us to see brain's response to pain, and the disparity attached to this response can be analyzed.[16]

As it is generally the case for all human experience, both injury and disease-related discomfort are more or less distinct from the experience of infrahuman beings. It seems unlikely that infrahuman species would experience sentience metaphorically. In contrast, if the human experience were to be described in a single word, that word would be "metaphoric." People experience their bodies symbolically. Verbal languages make frequent references to the symbolism of our bodies. We speak of irritants as being a "pain in the neck" or "in the back." We speak of emotional burdens as if they were physical and we say "oh, my aching back." In addition, it has long been noted that people are more likely to experience discomfort in places in their bodies that correspond to their mental attitudes in some metaphoric manner. Of course, physical pain is always real, whatever its connection with psychological issues.

No matter how tenuous the foregoing idea may sound, the body of reliable objective evidence in support of it is substantial. Formal investigations of psychological substrata of diseases thought to be physical are infrequent, however physical illness investigated to date demonstrates important psychological causes. The conclusion seems inescapable that particular psychological causes manifest in particular parts of the body according to a pattern best understood metaphorically. Of course, as far as we know, infrahuman animals are more or less beyond metaphor, and their physical manifestations are not known to resonate with their emotional histories. Sussman and Ferguson demonstrated that a lasting impact of aversive experience in rats had a lasting impact on rats who showed no evidence of retained learning due to their young age at the time of the experience.[17] Evidence of this impact is reflected in physical manifestations such as bolus counts. Perhaps this is an evolutionary precursor to the metaphoric experience of the body. Nonetheless, it falls far short of the kind of experience which is the general case for humans.

Whatever claims are made for animal awareness, it is clear that verbal metaphor is uniquely human. It is generally accepted among psychotherapists that the particular language individuals use in describing their experience can be especially meaningful.

THE MANIFESTATIONS OF PAIN

Yes, pain is terrible. In order to help you, your medical team will be interested in your description of pain, so you will want to take notes during the day and even at night to help you to communicate with your medical team members. When does the pain happen? How long does it last? Which adjectives will you use to describe it? Is it a type of pain new or did you have this pain in the past? Is the intensity the same as in the past? When and where does the pain start in a specific day? When and where does it end? What does the pain keep you from doing? What do you do to fight the pain? Does it stop you from moving, walking, climbing stairs, bathing, working, playing, breathing properly, eating, laughing, coughing, picking up and hugging your child (one of us solved this one by putting the toddler on the stairs to the same height as the arms)? What makes the pain better? What makes it worse? Many things relieve pain for some but are useless to other people. What did you try without any positive effects? Oftentimes the patterns inherent in these matters are meaningful.

> *Pain may continue unabated until the end. Pain, then, is more than an intriguing puzzle. It is a terrible problem that faces all humanity.*
>
> Melzack, 1973, p. 20.

The experience of pain raises questions of cause and effect: does the pain stop you from driving because it interferes with thinking and concentration? Or, could it be that your driving has somehow become aversive to you and having pain provides a means to stop doing it? Does it interfere with being close to other people because they do not care about you and do not understand? Or is it possible that you are avoiding intimacy through having pain? Does pain bring you to tears or do you feel tearful when you think of your pain? These are very common problems associated with the experience of chronic pain. Does pain interrupt your sleep? Does it change your mood? Does it affect your appetite and how?

When pain interacts with sleep, mood and appetite, it can affect all parts of life. Lack of sleep can become a major issue because without sleep, you have less energy to work, care for your family, manage your pain, enjoy life and do the things which are important to you. Pain can change the way you eat and cause you to gain or lose weight. Permanent pain will affect how you feel emotionally with a wide range of possibilities including depression and anger. Of course, your emotional state can easily affect your family, too. The psychological impact of chronic pain can change the way you feel about yourself and others.

The emergence of new pain often causes worry and concern. New pain does not necessarily mean that something is wrong because it can be caused by treatments or not moving around. Staying in the same position can be good for someone but very bad for another person. It may have mixed effects, allowing part of the body to rest and heal while depleting muscle tone and strength.

Although it is sometimes possible to find tissue damage at the site of pain, most of the time the case of pain is physically invisible. It should be added that pain falsification (malingering), for instance for insurance purposes, is very rare. Your physician (or any other health care professional whose training encourages a focus upon the physical to the exclusion of other domains) may doubt whether the pain is real. For this reason, it is very important to know the answers to the questions that we have just listed.

Perhaps in part due to an impoverished understanding, there has been a proliferation of diagnostic terms making reference to various conditions reported to be associated with unremitting pain, including chronic fibromyalgia, fibrositis, myofascial pain, chronic pain syndrome, chronic fatigue syndrome, myalgic encephalomyelitis, nonarticular rheumatism, psychogenic rheumatism, post-traumatic stress disorder, repetitive strain injury, sympathetic-mediated pain. These conditions have in common persistent soft tissue pain, an obscure relationship to a specific injury, and an obscure mechanism producing the experience of pain and illness.[18] Several of the above names are used for the same condition and this can become very confusing for the one with pain.

CHALLENGES IN TREATING PAIN

Pain is as difficult to treat as it is to define. Different kinds of pain respond to different treatment; you should know what has been tried and what you are now doing to manage your pain. Perhaps you also have ideas about what you would like to try in future. What works for one person may not work for the next; and no one really knows in advance how painkillers will affect any one person. The precise mechanisms of medication action often are not well known. You should be able to describe how long the medication takes to work and how long the pain relief, if any, lasts. Does the pain return before the next dose is due?

Are you willing to increase doses? Or would you prefer to decrease them? These are other questions to answer and discuss with your physicians.

Apt treatment of pain involves a multi-disciplinary team of caregivers and a multi-modal approach. One does well to be prepared to answer questions repeatedly because of the number of people in your medical team and because there will be different written forms to complete along the way. We know it is very frustrating to encounter the same lengthy questionnaire repeatedly when you are in pain. However your healthcare providers do not exchange information without your consent and you are the central point managing your treatment and communicating with your team members. Your general physician will want you to answer questions, so assessing your pain and describing it are necessary. Other team members will have much the same questions, for instance your chiropractor or massage therapist or physiotherapist. It is even more important to ask and answer questions if you have allergies or experience medication side effects.

Biologically, chronic pain is a signal of harm to the body. Psychologically, chronic pain may create emotional suffering. Behaviorally, chronic pain often causes alteration in former patterns of movements. Cognitively, chronic pain commonly occupies our mind with thoughts of causes and possible solutions. Spiritually, chronic pain is a reminder of our vulnerability. Culturally, chronic pain is viewed differently depending upon tradition.[19] It is very important to build a team caring for you and looking at your challenges with the same glasses as yours, a team having affinities with you. This team extends the pain threshold (the point when pain appears) and also increases the pain tolerance (the amount of pain we can take). Of course you are the one to set realistic goals and look after your health, as you will read. But you will require support and care from a team of professionals because of the complexity of chronic pain. You will decide who should be on your team and you will work in partnership with your healthcare providers. However even if you listen to them and receive advice, you will be the key person to make decisions on your treatment.

THE MANY FACES OF PAIN

The most common type of pain is referred to as nociceptive pain. Nociceptive pain follows when the pain receptors, called nociceptors, send signals to the brain via neuronal pathways located in the spinal column. This pain serves to inform us of a danger as we are able to take measures to protect ourself or prevent further injury. Arthritis, several kinds of neck and back pain, muscle or bone injuries pain, osteoporosis pain, some kinds of cancer pain, pressure from an injection or surgery are nociceptive pain. It may be experienced as sharp, dull or aching, in a small or large or multiple areas. Usually it goes away as the damage to the body heals. However nociceptive pain can last for months, years, or a lifetime (i.e., when the damaged tissues do not heal or when chronic inflammation is involved).

A second type of pain, neuropathic pain, is caused by injuries to nerves or other changes in the nervous system. The disturbed nervous system sends pain signals to the brain even when there is no other ongoing tissue damage. Neuropathic pain may be experienced as tingling, aching or burning and it can last for months, years or a lifetime. This pain is very difficult to manage. It appears and disappears for no apparent reason, and can also become permanent with various degrees of intensity. I find this form of pain to be the most annoying type of pain for me. It is a sort of sunburn close to the skin and difficult to ignore. Most pain killers are unable to treat this pain. Cold showers are useful, at least for me. This pain can burn and hurt so much that sometimes rolling in the snow seems to be the best treatment. It is exhausting and often too widely spread to be treated locally with acupressure points. Massages can be a sort of torture and don't provide immediate benefit. Even exercises, heat or cold pads seem to increase this pain.

Another form of neuropathic pain is phantom limb pain. This occurs when a person who has had an arm or leg removed continues to experience pain as if it were coming from the missing limb. The disturbed nervous system sends pain signals to the brain where they are interpreted as coming from a part of the body that no longer exists. Other kinds of neuropathic pain are trigeminal neuralgia, peripheral neuropathy, postherpetic neuralgia (shingles) and complex regional pain syndrome.

A third type of pain is called idiopathic pain, this means that the cause is unknown. Many people with chronic pain experience this form of pain as doctors are unable to discover the reason for it.

THE PAST AND PRESENT SCIENCE OF PAIN

Examples of pain are found in literature as early as the ancient Greek writings with Philoctetes suffering from chronic pain caused by a snake bite; his companions at the time of the Trojan war abandoned him on a deserted island because his cries of pain never stopped day or night, but the gods ordered them to go back to get Philoctetes and care for him. Abandoning the ill appeared to be immoral in Greek society and this can be extended to any civilizations. In my experience the science of pain has not changed much since the Trojan wars when "herbs gathered from the earth's floor" were used to soothe pain; we are still looking for a cure 2, 500 years after Sophocles' birth. Until the mid-seventeenth century, doctors believed that all pain was felt in the heart. However René Descartes, the philosopher and scientist, developed the idea of pain pathways with nerves going to the brain. This concept was wonderfully advanced for its day.[20]

> No one to
> Care for him! Always
> Racked with pain,
> Pain forever
> Eating at him, eating,
> Eating!...
> Bereft of all life's
> Gifts! Cast out;
> Alone;...
> No peace for his thoughts! No
> Cure for his fear! Only
> Echo babbling some
> Distant reply from the
> Hills to his endless
> Round of cries!
> Pity him!
>
> Chorus about Philoctetes,
> Sophocles, 496 - 406 B.C.

Role played by nerves

Usually pain sensory nerves serve as a system responding to temperatures and trauma. Pain involves processes taking place in the pheripheral tissues, such as nerve irritation, muscle spasm, inflammation. There are two types of sensory nerve fibers carrying the pain message to the spinal cord: A-delta fibers carry the message to the spinal cord at about 40 miles per hour and C fibers carry the message at approximately 3 miles per hour. Pain nerves are stimulated by very hot or cold temperatures, trauma or chemicals released during inflammation. These sensory nerves bring information about pain to the spinal cord by passing the sensations to other nerve cells in the spinal cord. Pressure can reduce some pain because the sensory nerve fibers, which carry pressure and touch messages to the spinal cord, are stimulated by pressure. These fibers are called A-beta fibers and they carry their message to the spinal cord at 180 – 200 miles per hour. Then they race to the spinal cord and override or at least compete with the incoming pain messages carried by the C and A-delta fibers.

If the calming impact of the A-beta fibers reaches the spinal cord before the pain messages carried by the other fibers, pain may be reduced if it is intense or not felt at all if it is mild. The concept involving the duration and frequency of a nerve's message, and competing nerve signals, all playing a role in nature and priority of information passed to the brain, is called the "gate control theory." This system was first proposed in 1965 by psychologist Ronald Melzack and anatomist Patrick Wall. It now appears that other factors, such as emotions, can both close and open the gates. This of course has enormous implications for the human condition. We now know that physical as well as psychological factors guide the brain's interpretation of painful sensations. For example, many athletes do not experience pain during intense activities.[21]

BRAIN: THE REAL SOURCE OF PAIN

Pain messages that reach spinal cord, encounter a very complicated system that sends, modifies again or cancels the message in its way to the brain. The thalamus routes pain signals to different parts of the brain and the anterior cingulate cortex governs the emotional response to pain.[22] Pain suppressors, such as serotonin and the endorphins (meaning endogenous morphine, the body's own natural opioid messengers), and numerous other chemicals are unleashed by the brain to inhibit or reduce the pain messages. So if we force these substances to develop by rubbing or exercising, and if we develop with pressure and rubbing the A-beta fibers altering the pain messages, we reduce, with the help from the A-beta fibers, the importance of the pain messages before they affect the brain. However chronic pain may also develop when a pain-sensing nerve is injured and sends out constant false-alarm signals to the brain, or when an injured pain nerve tries to regenerate because abnormal nerve conditions prevent the nerve from regulating pain level.

In addition, the body's ability to reduce pain messages may be compromised if the pain system itself is injured or if the spinal cord is bombarded with persistent and intense pain signals.[23] Some people with chronic pain exhibit greater brain activity than healthy people when subjected to pain. This may explain why they experience pain more severely.[24] On the other hand, pain appears to leave a cellular memory that sensitizes the spinal cord, making subsequent pain worse.[25] Another reason for intense chronic pain is the fact that some people with chronic pain may lose the ability to block incoming pain messages, so signals are uncontrolled and pain of once harmless sensations is magnified.[26] If the brain sends a message back down to close the gate, the pain signals to the brain are blocked. If the brain orders the pain gates to open wider, the pain signals intensify. When people are depressed, negative feelings may open the gate. However the gate theory appears now to provide only a partial explanation because

thoughts and emotions can directly influence physiological responses, for example muscle tension, playing a role
in the production of pain.[27] Pain raises questions of cause
and effect that have no singular or final answer. So, please,
develop working answers and be open for other answers
tomorrow. Then you can't be wrong.

Pain and injury are coexistent. Have you noticed how
we tend to see connected with pain anything that is wrong
in our lives? We don't have a busy social calendar? The
cause of it is the pain! We can't afford to travel or drive a
Porsche? The reason is the pain! Then, what about the ones
who have spinal injuries and drive a Porsche? Of course
chronic pain has a major impact on all aspects of life but
it is always possible to bring changes to reduce this effect,
instead of blaming our pain.

Researchers are currently trying to isolate genes associated with pain and recently studies conclude that gender
and hormones play roles in the domain of pain. Women
tend to report more severe and persistent pain than men.
Women also experience less pain when they have more
estrogen and this means pain is felt differently according
to the time in menstrual cycles.[28] Some painkillers are also
more effective on women than men. Some current studies
seem to show that two proteins in the brain trigger the
neuronal changes that amplify and sustain chronic pain
and medications inhibiting these proteins may help reduce
chronic pain. The brain not only receives pain signals from
the spinal cord but also seems to undergo changes in the
neuronal connections. These changes would be key to the
development of chronic pain. Therefore managing pain
remains a challenge which cannot be relieved by standard
medications.[29] Pain must be taken seriously because it may
even cause the body to develop an immune system defi-

ciency caused by the continual challenges that the body faces in combating it.

Pain is different from suffering because pain is a more physical sensation, while suffering is emotional reaction to pain. One goal is to experience pain without suffering in order to maintain quality of life. Pain is a symptom that may become a disease (for example, when it is chronic and does not go away). When pain becomes a disease, it is very difficult to manage because the brain's perception of pain keeps increasing: the syndrome caused by pain causes further pain. This phenomenon is called "cycle of pain."[30] It is a vicious circle. The good thing about vicious circles is that anything that interferes with them reduces their effect.

Controlling muscles helps to reduce pain from muscle spasms and tension. The muscles become tight and painful as a result of reflexive guarding of a painful area, nerve irritation or a generalized tension response. The brain is the final and powerful judge making decisions on pain. The brain responds to the strength, repetitiveness and duration of the pain message created by normal or calming or abnormal pain nerves. The brain can fire impulses to release endorphins and other pain relieving substances. It can also transform the pain message into a painful conscious experience for good or for ill. The brain can sometimes reverse a vicious cycle, making it auspicious.

The phenomenon of pain remains complex because it involves signals related to tissue injury or condition, but also our reactions to these signals. When we know pain comes from the brain, we try to develop physical and mental resilience and we understand the impor-

> **The brain gives meaning to the pain message.**
> Caudill, 1995, p. 26 - 27.

tance of negotiating and talking to the brain which is our friend or our enemy in a life long relationship.

Because we bind time and because our sentience is metaphoric by nature, we human beings are vulnerable to developing chronic physical manifestations of our emotional pain. These physical manifestations can come in the form of aches and pain for which there may be no objective medical evidence. In contrast to this, they can manifest so powerfully that tissue is in fact physically affected, and medical findings are positive. In addition, they can take the form of focal disturbances in immune function, disrupting our normally strong resistance to the myriad of allergens, pathogens, and environmental irritants and toxins we encounter every day. We also invent things like cars that wind us up with injuries that won't exactly heal on their own, and frequently become chronic. In this second case, the injuries and the pains and the metaphors interact.

THE DEFINITION OF PAIN FE 8 - 11 , 2011

The meaning of pain goes from discomfort to the following sentence:

> "a pain state in which the cause of the pain cannot be removed or otherwise treated and which in the generally accepted course of medical practice, no relief or cure of the cause of pain is possible or none has been found after reasonable efforts including, but not limited to, evaluation by the attending physician and surgeon and one or more physicians and surgeons specializing in the treatment of the area, system or organ

of the body perceived as the source of the pain."[31]

Of course pain is complex and is divided into acute pain when a cause is obvious and pain fades away, and into chronic pain when pain lasts more than 6 months or a reasonable time period. Pain can start as a symptom and quickly become a disease. We will show that even if chronic pain cannot be cured, it can be managed and healed; the ones with chronic pain can have a certain quality of life with appropriate care and support. A cure is a significant decrease of the physical issues while healing brings relief even if suffering is still present. Healing pain is possible even if a cure is often impossible.

Pain and horrific numbers

The facts concerning the incidence and impact of pain are painful to write or read. Well over 90 million North Americans suffer from chronic pain but figures are difficult to obtain because the conditions causing pain are numerous and complex. Pain causes more disabilities than cancer and heart disease combined.[32] Each year up to 15 million Europeans consider suicide because of chronic pain.[33] Surveys indicate over 18% of Canadians experience severe levels of chronic pain. For many, this pain is disabling. This means that several million people in the country experience chronic pain. At any given moment, half of all Canadians will have experienced some kind of pain in the past two weeks. A majority of Canadians experience head pain at least monthly.[34] About 30% of people in the US suffer from chronic pain and in Britain the most common symptom treated by doctors is headache.[35]

The problem is staggering. Because the very nature of pain spans many medical horizons, the extent of the problem is difficult to quantify. Add to this that people who do not seek medical help are not represented in statistics. The Canadian Migraine Association reports that almost 3.2 million Canadians over the age of 15 suffer from migraine. This figure represents 17% of the population, excluding children. Wells calculated that in North America over 26 million people suffer from migraine headaches.[36] As many as 15 % of Canadians suffer from lower back pain. Arthritis, an inflammation of joints, affects one in six Canadians and 37 million North Americans. The problem is far from being isolated.[37]

Pain is a silent epidemic that will spread even more because of our aging population. Data collected from 1008 persons with pain in 2004 in Canada indicate that 24% report constant pain, 49% have daily pain, the ones with osteoarthritis reporting the highest degree of constant pain (42%) followed by individuals with rheumatoid arthritis (30%). These figures were recently released by the Canadian Pain Coalition.

Unfortunately people who have chronic pain generally do not receive adequate treatment. The tragedy is that much pain-related suffering is unnecessary. As much as 90% of pain of any terminal illness can be controlled with medication.[38] Over 70% of people with cancer, for example, experience moderate to severe pain during their illness, yet fewer than half of them receive adequate analgesic treatment.[39] According to data reviewed by the Chronic Pain Association of Canada, a study at one large medical center found that the majority of hospital clients who were in substantial pain were not even asked by their doctors or nurses if they were experiencing pain. Most chronic pain symptoms go untreated even though effective relief through medication is available, and a good multi-disciplinary recovery pain team could certainly be used to reduce or eliminate these symptoms. Many people in pain allow their discomfort to take over their life, and even basic activities which people without pain take for granted, represent major challenges to those in pain. As a consequence, people in pain may find it difficult to communicate with people who do not have chronic pain.

The medical system often fails in treating people with pain because the underlying causes of pain are ignored. Tranquilizers are commonly prescribed for chronic pain although these medications do not directly decrease pain, and the neurological aspects of pain are not always addressed even though chronic pain alters brain function. Pain mobilizes neurons spread in four key zones of the brain and enervating the entire physical body, to vital functions, such as blood pressure and heart, and to emotions.[40]

Unfortunately our health care system does not always compensate many family doctors for pre and post service time to review records of previous treatments and develop a formal care plan. Therefore many receive inadequate treatment. In addition, the way people spend their pain management money should be reviewed because we tend to deal first – and sometimes only – with injuries that are visible, such as a disjointed jaw or a broken bone. Quite often no money is invested on what would reduce invisible issues causing pain, such as stress and lack of relaxation. We recommend to spend 50% of our pain management budget on treating medically proven and visible injuries and we suggest to use the remaining money on reducing the invisible causes of pain. Unfortunately our current environment does not really help us to make this type of decisions. We live in a country where we are closer to a national policy on euthanasia than to one on pain relief providing guidelines protecting physicians and clients alike.[41]

It is not surprising that pain is devastating to individuals and families. When pain persists, it becomes part of the fabric of life, often making it difficult to concentrate, remember and to perform even routine tasks. Lost workdays and medical costs can easily become financially ruinous. Lack of revenues combined with increased expenses makes it difficult for families where members experience chronic pain. The person with pain then feels guilty. Reduced revenues become a burden affecting relationships between spouses because it is difficult for the one who is not in physical pain to understand the need for these expenses. One of the most common reasons people buy books on suicide and support physician-assisted suicide is a fear of intractable pain. This fear of aging with pain is another topic that spouses find difficult to share. Pain goes hand in hand with lack of sleep and depression.

NEEDLESS PAIN

Too many children in pain: a shame in our society

Of course, pain can also be a tragedy for children and their families. Our understanding that pain touches children and teenagers is recent and incomplete. Younger people and newborns have a right to be treated humanely and effectively for pain. However this right was not taken into consideration up to a few years ago. Even as recently as the 1980s, it was believed infants did not feel pain. To this horrible myth were added a lack of tools for the assessment of pain among newborns, fears about side effects from medications and numerous other wrong beliefs, such as "pain builds characters" or "they will grow out of it" when referring to conditions causing childhood pain. Therefore acute, chronic or recurrent pain suffered by infants and children on each continent was very often not treated. Blood samples, immunization and circumcision used to be done without pain relievers. Until the mid 1980s newborns were also routinely operated in Northern America with paralyzing agents making them unable to move but allowing them to feel pain.[42]

However in 1987 Dutch doctors started to challenge the belief newborns did not feel pain and slowly the rest of the world modified their common beliefs. An international study has just proven newborns are highly sensitive to pain and may be more vulnerable to its long term consequences than older children and adults. The same research also concluded that hormonal, metabolic and cardiovascular responses to surgery were more pronounced in newborns than older children. We know now that a foetus can feel pain as early as the 26th week of pregnancy.[43]

Why did no one challenge this shameful myth that newborns do not feel pain? Most probably because infants have no political power and can't lobby for their pain. Many caregivers were also taught that newborns do not feel pain. In late 1989 I was expecting one of my two daughters and, having a critical pregnancy, I was admitted to the best western Canadian hospital for prenatal medicine. The goal was to take a blood sample from the baby or from the part of the cord holding the baby's blood, in order to confirm the amniocentesis results. Well, only by looking, on the ultrasound screen, at the 5 month not yet born baby, I knew she was feeling a form of pain and danger. When the needle came close to her, she would kick it with her feet to protect her body and she would flip over quickly before going away as far as possible to the other side of the uterus. My medical team (and of course myself who decided to stop the "procedure") concluded the baby was normal because of her quick flight reaction in front of an object entering her protected world; it was impossible to take the blood sample because she moved away too fast from the needle. After birth, tests confirmed she was normal, healthy and very intelligent. This dramatic experience opened my eyes on numerous ethical and medical issues; in 1989 it convinced me babies felt stress and pain even before birth.

> Baby mine, don't you cry, let your life sparkle and shine, baby mine.
>
> Walt Disney,
> Dumbo's mother singing to her disabled baby in pain.

Assessing intensity of children's pain

So, why did it take until 1987 for science to challenge the assumption infants did not feel pain? We can find several reasons but the fact that infants' cries do not tell us where it hurts, how much and which type of pain they have, seems to remain the most common excuse for the initial inattention to pain among newborns. It is true several methods of assessing pain among young children exist, such as studying their facial expressions, their cries and limb movements or asking them to select a face between a series of faces going from tears to smiles. The assumption is the child will pick up the face best matching his or her mood. Children can explain how they feel by comparison with other painful situations such as falling from a bike or being stung by a mosquito. I like to use this method because it provides a distraction by referring to other past events that can be related to solutions followed for their previous experiences. Another way to assess the intensity of pain is to ask for its size going from a pea to an apple. However no objective method to measure pain exists for anyone, regardless of age. This lack of scientific clinical tools still causes young children's pain not to be taken very seriously. How frustrating for parents and caregivers!

In adults and children alike, it is now accepted that pain slows learning and reduces sleep and appetite. It is also suspected that pain places young children at risk of developing a dysfunctional pain defense system in adulthood.[44] Children tend to dramatize and develop fears regarding what they are unable to understand. Untreated pain can then cause anxiety. According to very recent research, infants who experience little pain, develop better health and behavior.

Too many kids in pain, not enough research

An estimated 10 million Americans 18 and younger in the United States suffer from chronic or recurrent pain; about one quarter of teenagers report headaches. Apparently the incidence of these conditions is increasing. Underlying causal conditions include headache, migraine, cancer, cystic fibrosis, musculoskeletal and nerve injury from accidents and fracture.[45] Abdominal pain (also fairly common among children and teen-agers) has a multitude of often poorly-defined possible causes. Research on treatment of chronic pain in children is extremely limited; and with our current health system suffering from lack of funding, this is unlikely to change. Pediatric pain clinics are expensive to run, and insurance rarely sufficiently compensates for so-called alternative treatments such as massage and psychology.[46]

Most mind-body interventions known to decrease pain among adults can be used with children, who have an even better imagination than adults and can easily be hypnotized with stories, games and videos. Because of their unlimited imagination and belief in magic, children trust the most unbelievable stories are real. It is not surprising then that mind-body techniques are very successful with them. Simple procedures, such as close contact with a parent or a pacifier with a sugar solution during painful routine procedures, are known to reduce infants' reaction to pain. Tender touch, combining kisses, hugs, massages, warm baths and stories, of course remains the first tool parents use in healing children. On the other hand, topical pain relievers (i.e. lidocaine) can be used during circumcision and acetaminophen can be given for postoperative pain. Even morphine and fentanyl can be given safely to newborns.[47]

Unfortunately the best pharmaceuticals and the right doses remain an issue because parents tend not to allow their children to be used in clinical trials. What parents could blame them? On the other hand, in Canada pharmaceutical companies finance medical research. As a result, experts are put in a difficult position when they provide objective results, and their reports are not available to everybody. This means regulators, physicians and parents don't have complete information on many medication effects.[48] Exact doses for many medications taken by children are often unknown and people still believe a little less is better than a little more because of the traditional view stating children will get used to a medication that will not work well at a later date when this same medication becomes really necessary. The familiar labels that indicate dose according to age rather than weight are often misleading as weight can be a better guideline than is age. Have you noticed how many 10 year-old children dress a size 7? And what about teen-agers who have an adult size even if they are still officially children for the age? The question of whether race makes a difference in selecting doses usually remains unaddressed. Many barriers prevent children from getting appropriate medications and doses. Good pediatricians or long term family physicians should be consulted because they have the experience of knowing past reactions to the same medications with other children. Parents can also judge some doses because of their experience with giving medication to their children.[49]

REASONS FOR UNDER-TREATING PAIN

A large number of persons of all ages with chronic pain do not see a doctor on a regular basis even if pain reduces their quality of life. Why? Some are scared because they believe the physician will discover a terrible illness, others believe enduring pain is heroic, while others believe pain is normal. Everybody has a reason, but as a consequence pain becomes seriously under-treated and statistics are never very accurate.

Another group of people who commonly experience under-treated pain is the elderly, who are expected to endure pain as normal part of their daily lives. This is also false. Totally wrong! Failure to assess pain, the inaccurate belief that pain treatments are

> *What can't be cured must be endured, is the very worst and most dangerous maxim for a nurse ever to be made. Patience and resignation in her are but other words for carelessness or indifference.*
>
> Florence Nightingale, nurse and writer, founder of universal health care, who experienced chronic pain.

less effective in the elderly, and the false belief that the elderly are less sensitive to pain provide additional explanations for under-treatment of pain among the elderly.[50] Unfortunately "pain contributes increasingly to physical dysfunction with older age"[51] when pain can be decreased even among the elderly who should be allowed to enjoy a good quality of life. Pain is not necessarily normal with aging.

On the other hand, pain is costly to society. The annual direct cost of chronic pain (including medical expenses, lost income and lost productivity, but no social costs) is estimated to exceed $10 billion in Canada. Lost workdays in North America resulting from chronic pain add up to well over 55 million a year.[52] The indirect cost is impossible to estimate but probably dwarfs the direct cost.

However most pain can be decreased. According to experts 90% of cancer pain can be relieved by relatively simple means. But fewer than half of people with cancer receive adequate treatment for pain. A recent survey in the Medical Post indicated that 55% of physicians in Canada felt their peers were not doing enough to treat cancer pain. Another survey of oncologists revealed that only 12% of those surveyed thought they received good to excellent training in pain management in medical school and only 27% gave a high rating for training during residency. Another study of neurologists indicated only 30% of practicing neurologists were "adequately trained to diagnose pain" and only 20% felt "adequately trained to treat the entire spectrum of pain disorders."[53] Most physicians and other healthcare professionals are simply not prepared, by education or training, to assist people in pain.

Most persons experiencing pain have little or no awareness that a safe, effective treatment is probably available for them. Therefore most pain is under-treated. One recent study of persons with chronic pain involved in litigation concluded that the overall rate of inaccurate or incomplete diagnosis at referral was 40% to 67%. In a large survey of oncologists, 86% of respondents felt that the majority of clients with pain were under-medicated.[54] In general the lack of medical training in pain management and the uneasiness of both healthcare providers and clients to deal with pain leads to the widespread under-treatment of both acute and chronic pain. Most physicians are reluctant to prescribe opioid analgesics because they believe their clients will become addicted or because they fear investigation and sanctions by regulatory bodies. The fear of giving opioids and causing addiction among clients is also connected to healthcare professionals' fear of being sued by clients because of possible side effects. So healthcare providers worry about litigation from regulatory bodies and clients. It is not surprising then if many prefer not to prescribe narcotics!

The following two realities could also be better represented in the medical management of pain: experiential and learned factors influence the immune response, and the physiological substrate of that influence is known, at least in part. The immune response is programmed by information from the central nervous system. Embryonic T-cells have been micrographed forming synaptic connections with neurons originating in the central nervous system. In addition, it has long been understood that opiates have their primary action in areas of the central nervous system mediating the sense of pleasure and reward. They create a sense of pleasure; they do not kill pain. It is unfortunate that the implications of this knowledge have not so far become the basis of a deeper understanding of pain management.

Politicians, regulators, health insurers and society at large lack also awareness and understanding of pain; this makes pain management even more difficult. Many insurance companies that face ever-increasing pressure to pay compensation often dismiss the one with pain as a malingerer. This may be due to the fact that objective measures of pain do not exist. Also, pain can be expensive to treat. Unfortunately insurance for car accidents and other injuries often create barriers to long term medical treatment by arguing about the legal legitimacy of claims related to pain. In addition, many people do not claim expenses from insurance when they need the funding necessary for aggressive treatment that can reduce long term suffering and prevent chronic pain. Why? Maybe they fear increased premiums. Perhaps they also lack information about possible treatments.

Numerous myths about pain surround us because invisible conditions such as pain are generally stigmatized by society. Therefore clients and healthcare professionals are embarrassed about pain and reluctant to acknowledge it. Society has led many people to believe they "must learn to live with it." We believe the days when we were told "I am sorry but you will have to learn to live with pain" must end forever. This passive attitude does not help people to develop strategies to decrease pain and suffering. If you go to the emergency room after a car accident, you will most probably be told you will have pain for a long time. It may not be explained that, even if there is pain for a long time or for ever, it is possible to control it. Unfortunately we are never told right away this control is possible and usually we only come to learn of it after years of pain.

Ironically persons experiencing pain are even part of

the problem because many believe pain is inevitable, that they must live with it and not complain. Some may have also a fear of becoming addicted to medication and of being unable to perform activities if they take painkillers. Some are also scared of side effects. Here I remember a few seniors who like to say: "No pain, no brain" and refuse to take painkillers for a long time while cancer and other painful conditions invade their body. It takes time to remove fears attached to side effects from medication even among the ones who are critically ill and in pain. It takes time to train people to believe everybody can benefit from psychotherapy and many cannot afford the fees charged for long time counseling.

Some people take less of their dosage than prescribed because of these fears. Others believe that, if they take painkillers early on, when the pain is bearable, painkillers will be less effective later when pain is more severe. Unfortunately most people in pain have little or no awareness that treatment, by a good caring doctor, for pain with medication combined with non-medication techniques is safe and effective, if followed properly, even if it takes time to find the best treatment. Most people do not know that many do not develop any significant tolerance and reach a plateau in what dosage they require, with some even able to lower their dosage as the pain becomes more controlled. In most cases there is nothing wrong with stronger doses if they improve quality of life and are part of a well managed plan that also includes psychotherapy and exercise.

Consequences for under-treating pain

Another myth about pain is that it is not lethal. However if you wear your body out from fighting pain, you divert your strength and resources for fighting the underlying disease. Unrelieved pain can also lead to suicide. According to statistics collected by the Chronic Pain Association of Canada, people with pain have a suicide rate 9 times greater than that of the general population. The most common reason for supporting physician-assisted suicide is the fear of intractable pain. In another survey, 69% of people with cancer reported that they would consider committing suicide if their pain was not treated adequately.[55] We know also that "relieving pain actually averts temporary, pain-related immune-system declines" which "have the potential to be life-threatening."[56] A research team at the University of California determined lab animals subjected to pain "were less capable of fighting the growth of cancerous tumors. Animals given injections of a pain killing medication were able to fight the tumors in a normal fashion."[57]

Some researchers today think also that the continued release of pain causing substances in chronic pain conditions leads to lasting nervous system changes which make some people hypersensitive to pain. These persons suffering with hyperalgesia can cry out in pain at the gentlest touch, or even if a soft breeze blows over the painful area. So, in effect good pain control should come at the beginning of a painful condition and not at the end.[58] Contrary to what many people and professionals think, the ones experiencing pain are not malingerers or hypochondriacs. Their activities are restricted. They are men, women and children of all ages, education and social background suffering with a wide spectrum of painful conditions which can be reduced and even disappear in many cases.

Healing is always possible

Many people do not make a difference between healing and curing. "Healed" represents a condition of one's life and "cured" relates strictly to one's physical condition. In other words there may be healed quadriplegics, dying people who are leading healthy lives, and cured people who had cancer and are leading unhealthy lives. This means that healing is always possible even with life-threatening diseases and even with chronic pain.[59] One physician who worked for the Cross Cancer Institute in Edmonton commented during a recent meeting how her dying clients could be healthy! In addition, an "illness" is not a "disease" which is a medical condition attached to a diagnosis. Of course the meaning of "healthy" and "healing" is very personal and can be defined only by you. Please do not see yourself as an ill person because illness does not apply to your entire person. We may be a person with a physical inconvenience or an illness or a physical disability. You make the distinction between these terms and you decide how you want to qualify chronic pain.

Our pain and the others

Each physician, healthcare professional and client should think about the meaning of words commonly used in the medical world. The word "care" has its roots in the Gothic *Kara*, meaning to grieve, experience sorrow, cry out with. The person who truly cares must join the person in pain.[60] Sometimes there is nothing else to do while the client tries to heal. Many physicians want so badly to fix people that they unfortunately are unable to be caregivers. The ones with chronic pain must be cured (if possible) but also, very importantly, healed and cared for. There is place for physicians and healers and in an ideal world, the same person would be physician and healer.

Sadly many people, even the caring ones, friends and family, do not always assist others in healing. Some of

AT PEACE WITH PAIN

them can be cruel even if they love you very much; others believe people create their own pain because of their attitude or mental condition. Who did not hear at least one time one of the following remarks? "I am afraid to hug you! You look so fragile!" Just what you need when you feel alone and lonely! "You seem to be doing so well!" This one is very common. It cuts any conversation before it even started! How could you reply you have pain? After all, no one asks you anything and everybody else feels better when there is no one suffering too closely. So, it becomes impossible to have a sincere conversation and communicate properly. "You look so slim! I envy you!" How could you say you do not eat properly because of pain in the jaws and mention you are too depressed to prepare a meal? "You are late! Your appointment was at 10:30, not 10:40 am!" This comment was heard from a chiropractor's receptionist. How could you say calmly the traffic is terrible, your neck hurts from cold weather and tension added to injuries? How could you say you pay this lady's salary and she should appreciate to see you at any time without becoming angry and hurting you even more? "You are smiling when you talk about your pain. You should be crying or complaining if you have so many problems." Who needs this type of comment? Crying could perhaps release tension and create a relaxation, by why complaining when complaining simply increases pain and depression? "You are ill because you did not find a good doctor. Try my physician if you want to recover." Of course we are all proud of our own doctors, but it may be really painful to be perceived as one unable to locate a good physician. It is also unfair to our own healthcare professionals trying their best. "You should be happy if you have only problems with muscles. At least you have no broken bone." True, but pain from

~ 49 ~

muscles can be very intense, even worse than childbirth pain. "At least you do not suffer from a degenerative disease." True, but hard to accept! Another one, very common with small differences, is this one: "Only people with a serious mental illness need a psychologist." After this statement, how do you explain you receive some relief from pain by healing your life thanks to a psychologist you see on a regular basis? How do you dare to explain to family and friends you are depressed and not crazy when you connect with a psychologist? "I never see a chiropractor! Do you know he could kill you by twisting your neck? It happened recently to someone! You should be more careful and not allow anyone to touch your neck." This one hurts a lot because you trust the person touching your neck, so it is not about death but about trust in someone who cares a lot for you. We heard these remarks many times, surprisingly often from other healthcare professionals.

So, we did our homework and discovered that chiropractors in Alberta spend about $700.00 per year on liability insurance when a neurologist can spend $25,000.00 per year for the same insurance. So, is a chiropractor likely to damage your neck when you look at the numbers? The risk of serious complications or death from manipulation of the cervical spine is 1 to 2 per million.[61] We also read that medical use of medications kills 100,000 persons in North America per year because of adverse reactions. This means about a jumbo jet crashing every day. Who cares for these 100,000 persons who die as a result of medications? Which newspapers report their death? According to Dr. Bruce Carleton of the University of British Columbia, medication complication would be one of the top 10 causes of death. Exact figures are unknown because the Food and Drug Administration in the U.S. and Health Canada depend on voluntary reports of adverse reactions. "How could you do so much, how could you work if you have so much pain?" We get this comment quite often from friends. We get it also from a few healthcare professionals ... but usually we do not go back to see them if they do not trust us and do not understand pain is real. How could they also understand that sometimes only the power of the mind keeps people going... especially people with young children needing protection? Otherwise, without power of mind, how could starving mothers carry their children to refugees' camps in Africa? "I finished the treatment! It went very well! Now it's up to your body to heal and you do not need me for now." Well, when one of us heard this one, we wondered what would happen if the body did not want to heal and pain did not go away. Where to go for support? We learned, since that time, there is always an open door somewhere. The challenge is to find it and to know where you could find someone to hug you. "After your day at the office, just go home and relax." We hear this one many times. Most parents have to work outside the home and care for children, including toddlers and teens. It is not easy to raise them with school, after school and social activities, sports ... and keeping a few hours a week for quality time with family. We hear the same comment, once in a while, even from friends, but we learned not to pay much attention to this type of advice. "Why do you invite all these children at home? You will become exhausted." How do you explain that these children and also our own kids keep us going and maintain a reason for us to heal? The first step of a good pain management program is to ignore these remarks and to realize these people love us even if they do not know how to say so.

OUR ITINERARY

Connection and transformation

Our goal in this book will be to show how to decrease pain and to heal lives. Both are essential to happiness. When we know more about pain, we already have less suffering because we become aware of various possible strategies. There is no miraculous way to cure chronic pain and for this reason, various approaches to pain management are offered in our book. Conventional and alternative medicine will be combined in our suggestions for an integrated pain management program. Alternative medicine is empowering and provides an ideal means to improve quality of life.[62] The best program integrates conventional medicine with alternative treatments of your choice to give you the best of both western and eastern worlds. We will work for peace of mind and taking charge of our life. We will also show how the diagnosis and management of chronic pain is a complex process requiring intensive, comprehensive and interdisciplinary services for the best outcomes.

The book will give an update on pain medication; it will insist on making connections as an essential element for healing; it will also cover other subjects and habits stimulating healing energy and making life better for the ones in pain. All these integrated approaches combine eastern and western medicine, scientific medicine as well as mind-body medicine and eternity or nonlocal medicine outside space and time. The book will allow you to explore different therapies and to decide for yourself which ones to follow.

Why a book about pain? Pain changed our life for ever and, so far, outside of short brochures and specialized publications not accessible to everybody, we have not found a book presenting a good comprehensive pain management plan giving options to the ones in pain, explaining advantages and disadvantages. Books on

> There is nothing final in the universe of mind or matter – all is tendency, growth.
>
> Florence Nightingale

pain written by people in pain for others in pain are more or less non-existent. This publication is a book of hope addressed to the ones who experience chronic pain, who need to heal their life, who have little or no support at all, who feel alone and lonely, who look for balance and harmony, who need unconditional love and who would like, just like us, to give a meaning to pain even if pain is needless. This book should remove misconceptions attached to pain and should prevent some additional suffering. Pain can be transformed into something positive; it helped us to discover connectedness and intimacy with wonderful people among other ones in pain, colleagues, family, friends, communities and healthcare professionals. Pain also allowed us to reach a closer connection with the universe, to develop a mission in life, to create beauty around us through the arts and to enjoy the present. Without all the people who taught us survival skills and shared freely, the book would have been impossible to write and we would have been unable to give a sense to our pain.

If this book helps you to select the right therapies among the medical, psychological, social and cultural models or to combine the best ones for you, if this book helps you to transform your pain into something less negative and to find a mission in life, we will have reached our goals.

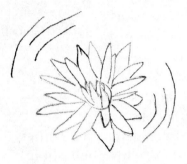

Chapter 2

MEDICATION

2:00 a.m. Sunburn pain on my neck and shoulders. Pulling and stretching pain on my face and neck. Pressing pain on my heart. Also stabbing pain between the shoulder blades and on the left hip. Constant ringing in the ears just like being surrounded by a swarm of bees. The splint between the jaws is another source of major discomfort. Impossible to sleep.

3:00 a.m. Outside birds start singing although it is still night. These melodies are a sign dawn is not very far. Better not to think how I'll feel tomorrow morning after another night without rest. Entire body stiff with pain winning and taking over. Headache more intense. It now seems a fountain is running in my head with this buzzing and tapping sound. I was told this is the noise produced by arteries bringing blood to the head, in all cases not a very reassuring explanation. Impossible to think clearly, so no need for explanations. Everything is very illogical. Impossible to find the right position to sleep. The back? Impossible to lie on a horizontal position because it increases the stabbing pain. Right side? No, it increases pain on the jaw and the right shoulder. Left side? No, it

crushes the shoulder. Even changing position is very dif-
ficult with a stiff body. On the stomach? Better not to
think about this one because impossible to turn head to
the right or left in order to breath. Feeling life is coming to
an end. Visualizing a parade of friendly faces. Trying to
concentrate on the images of spring flowers. Visualizing a
walk in the garden. For each comforting image, a stabbing
blow in the neck. Trying to review pain relief techniques,
but impossible to even breath deeply. It makes a major
difference to be alone at night at home and to be with a
coach encouraging you to fill up the lungs with air and
practice pain relief techniques. Pain increases even more
at the idea everybody else is resting peacefully. Last time I
looked at the red numbers on the clock, I read 3:45 a. m.
Medication helped to fall into a sort of dark hole which
passes for sleep.

Pain relief techniques may be directed toward conscious processes or toward the subconscious part of our minds. The techniques directed toward the conscious part of our minds generally relieve the physiological part of pain. They include medication, physical relief from ice or heat, and exercise. These techniques are traditionally taught in medical schools and have been medically researched. Other techniques, which are not usually included in traditional medical training, target the mind-body connection through the subconscious and attempt to relieve the suffering component of pain. They can be very important methods for managing chronic pain, and include muscle relaxation, distraction, meditation, yoga and hypnosis, biofeedback, acupuncture and acupressure.[1] Some of these techniques bring healing by strengthening the connection between conscious and unconscious parts of the mind. Specifically they induce altered states of consciousness.

MANY TYPES OF MEDICATION

Medications used in treating pain include a wide variety of families with analgesics, tricyclic antidepressants, anti-convulsants, muscle relaxants, opioids (also called "narcotics"), steroidal and non-steroidal anti-inflammatories. The analgesics include numerous medications. It is probably fair to say that the very abundance of pharmaceutical interventions indicates that there is no uniformly effective medication treatment for pain. As a result, selecting proper painkillers is difficult because different root causes and types of pain have a higher response rate to different medications and combinations of medications.

A major category of interest to those of us seeking pain relief is the non-steroidal anti-inflammatories (NSAIDS) including Aspirin ®, ibuprofen and also medications containing acetaminophen. Analgesics can be classified in three categories according to availability: the first level includes Aspirin ®, acetaminophen, ibuprofen and other NSAIDS. These are widely used as over the counter (OTC) preparations. The second level includes mild opioids such as codeine or oxycodone. The third level includes morphine and other morphine-related opioids. The last two levels are subject to strict legal control to prevent misuse and redirection to the street level. Marijuana, is slowly being recognized and is said to bring good results for some users. The active ingredient of marijuana (THC) is available by prescription and must be obtained by a compounding pharmacy in your area. However smoking is hazardous; getting a high is not recommended, but prudent use can be very effective and continues to be studied. Some healing agents found in marijuana are available in other countries by prescription under another form, such as a spray; it is hoped these alternative ways of accessing this medication will soon be available to all in Canada. Medication works either by interacting at the site of discomfort or by interacting with brain chemistry to reduce or neutralize the pain-producing substances of the brain and to replace them with comfort-producing substances. Medication can also stimulate the parts of the brain responsible for pleasure, allowing the body to relax. Opioids decrease pain by latching onto specific receptors on the outside of cells in the brain and elsewhere.[2] The experience of chronic pain taught me a lot about a number of medications and I know now there is no magic pill for everyone. Being comforted is an useful adjunct to healing. Properly used medications can and do provide comfort.

ASPIRIN® AND ACETAMINOPHEN

Folk remedies for pain have long included salicylate obtained from poplar tree, willow bark and a few other plants. The commercial production of sodium salicylate started around 1880 and about 1899 Bayer developed a medication it labelled Aspirin® ("a" for acetyl, "spir" from a plant containing salicin and "in" because this was a popular suffix). This new product became the leading medication for pain and as of 1915 was available over the counter. Although arguably the most familiar analgesic, research continues to demonstrate new and effective uses for Aspirin®, many of which do not include pain control. The major disadvantage of Aspirin® is the gastric upset and stimulating asthmatic conditions. When children use

Aspirin®, there is in addition a risk of developing Reye's syndrome, a potentially lethal form of liver failure. Aspirin® can also damage cartilage. Bones do not touch because the cartilage acting as a sponge, absorbing and holding water, provides a cushion within the joint. Aspirin® slows down this absorption and may cause joints to hurt even more, in addition to causing gastrointestinal irritation and bleeding.[3]

A new pain medication appeared for sale in 1960 under the name of acetaminophen which is now known as Tylenol®. This is not an anti-inflammatory medication but has the advantage of relieving pain without irritating the stomach. It can be suspended in liquid form which can be easily administered to babies and children.[4] We still do not understand how acetaminophen works.[5] Tylenol®'s most serious known disadvantage is potential damage to the liver and the kidney if taken in large doses (1000 – 1500 mg per day) over a long period of time.[6] This can ultimately lead to acetaminophen toxicity and liver failure if left unchecked.

The night I had the car accident, I went to the hospital. The doctor who examined me and checked my neck, said I was fine to go home. He added I should take something for pain, and warned me I would have pain for a long time. I asked him if I should take Aspirin ® since the "something" was fairly vague to me. He replied Tylenol® would be better. Now I know chronic use of Tylenol® can damage liver and kidneys.[7] I did not know it at the time and I took many of them while wondering what "a long time" could mean. Now I also know it could mean a life-time. You wouldn't want to use Tylenol® regularly during a life-time. Liver damage often does not repair itself.

ANTI-INFLAMMATORIES

Inflammation and pain go together. By reducing inflammation, it is possible to reduce pain. In the 1960s scientists began experimenting with a chemical compound called ibuprofen. Trials of a new medication called Motrin® and made of ibuprofen started in 1969 on people with certain types of arthritis. Results were very promising not only with arthritis but also with numerous other pains including pulled muscles and sore throats.[8] It took until the early 1970s when scientists discovered how anti-inflammatories work to reduce pain.

Anti-inflammatories have limitations in the treatment of chronic pain and can cause gastric irritation when taken orally on an empty stomach. I tried them as pills and as cream but I cannot say they made a difference to my pain even though my physicians believed they were going to help. Creams were enjoyable because of massages I performed on my arms and neck. I stopped using anti-inflammatories fairly quickly because they did not reduce my pain and were not the solution for me. I took them because my family doctor at the time was very positive about them and believed they would help. I took them to make my doctor happy. I wanted to be a good client.

DEEP INJECTIONS, IMPLANTS AND SURGERY

Invasive and aggressive therapies should only be followed once less extreme methods failed to relieve pain. In our experience these techniques are more promising in theory than in practice. Physicians offer to stimulate or medicate the spinal cord, coat nerves with anesthetic or steroids, or even kill these nerves. An injection of anesthetic and anti-inflammatory steroids can be administered under local anesthetic and the procedure is performed with the assistance of an imaging technique called fluoroscopy. This means the doctor can watch a video of your spine, nervous tissue or joint where the needle is being directed. In the procedure for nerve ablations, a pain-generating nerve is destroyed by freezing or heating. The nerve is then killed and not only numbed. The client receives a local anesthetic and the doctor introduces a thin wand to conduct cold or heat into the nerve site. At best pain disappears for about one year. Nerve ablations are not performed when a person has multiple painful sites because it is dangerous to kill too many nerves. In extreme cases of chronic pain, implanted pumps can be installed to deliver a strong medication, such as morphine, into the spinal cord. The pump removes the feeling of being heavily medicated because the medication does not pass through the digestive system.[9]

My own experience with injections was a magnificent disaster. I tried multiple injections in the muscle knots and the trigger points for only a few months. The procedure was fairly painful, especially in the neck and on the back of the head just above the neck. Posture was an issue; I sat on a chair to allow needles on the back of the head and neck.

The physician administering the shots was a very nice and compassionate man. He was sincerely sorry his treatment did not decrease my pain and stop muscle spasms. He then referred me to another physician, in the same clinic, who specialized in deep injections into the joint. This second treatment scared me when I understood the

procedure had to be done at the hospital in case complications arise. The plan was to freeze the skin on the neck,
use a sort of sophisticated X ray machine to view the area
to treat on a video and inject a painkiller/anti-inflamma-
tory into the surface of a joint on the neck (the C2-C3). I
decided to allow the procedure because it was promising
with a good rate of success according to a limited research
I did in published sources.

The treatment was scheduled to take place in a Edmonton
hospital. So I went for a first injection. A radiologist and
two nurses assisted the pain specialist. Yes, the procedure
was scary. The pain specialist inserted a needle to indicate on the screen the place where he wanted to inject the
analgesic. Conversation between the team members doing
the treatment was also very technical and they all seemed
fascinated by the "site" they were going to "treat" and did
not really pay attention to me as a person. In a sense, they
ignored me while they were watching a part of my body
on the screen. No one held my hand. They kept telling me
not to move and frankly I was scared to move because I
was worried about moving involuntarily and getting the
injection into the wrong place. I imagined the needle hit-
ting the spinal cord and I saw myself paralyzed from the
neck down. People had told me many times not to allow a
chiropractor to touch my neck. The injection seemed a lot
more dangerous than chiropraxis. The injection was not
too painful (certainly less painful than in my mind) and I
was happy to learn I could still walk. I had to rest for 30 mn
in a recovery room and while on the bed, my neck became
very stiff with no explanation from anyone. I heard the
treatment was very experimental. After the fact, I was told
by the pain specialist he did not want anyone, especially
a chiropractor, touching my neck even if my chiropractor

was a man I really trusted.

The "site" they "treated" burned a lot. I was released from the hospital and returned to work. Driving was difficult because of the stiff neck, which remained so for several days. The following week, just as my range of movement started to improve, I went back for the second injection. I sat in the waiting room before seeing the pain specialist. Then, it was my turn: I went in and sat in the client's chair in the room where I had received a first injection in the previous week.

The pain specialist saw how stiff I was and decided not to administer a second injection. He also told me there was nothing more to do for my neck to improve. Of course I started to cry... a lot. Then the pain specialist gave me a prescription for some medication which was supposed to help me. I took the piece of paper and left. I stopped crying in the car because I had to drive back to the office. I took the pain specialist's medication for a few days and did not care to know what they were. I believe they were an anti-inflammatory or a painkiller of some sort but cannot be certain. I did not even care to know what they were. I felt depressed for a long time. One should never leave a physician's office with this crushing pain of hopelessness.

> The bottom line was that she had a life of chronic pain ahead of her. In my view this just isn't good enough. That is why we need more pain research. We need new treatments for pain.
>
> Lynch, 2003, p. 63.

Below are a few myths and facts about medication that I have learned from my personal experience with chronic pain and have verified with research in scientific medical publications.

MYTHS AND FACTS

Myth: Painkillers have horrible side effects. Yes, they have side effects like any other medication. However your pain specialist will guide you and change them if necessary. Many side effects can be managed: A medication causing drowsiness can be taken at bedtime. Additional glasses of water are recommended if the medication causes dry mouth. Constipation, which is another side effect, can be managed with a diet rich in fibers and consuming large amounts of water with a stool softener. Liquorice and cashew nuts are also excellent snacks to help relieve constipation. Opioids are compatible with many other medications treating their side effects. Occasionally users may not experience side effects after using opioid medication for a few days. In my personal experience, opioids did not cause mental impairment and did not interfere with my mental abilities. I suspect this is because I take them with cautious mindfulness. Medications have an effect on the body, however the mind controls the body. The essential is to proceed mindfully.

Myth: Painkillers decrease your ability to function and concentrate and they will make you look medicated. The fact is that in appropriate doses, painkillers do not generally have an impact on the mind. If one causes adverse reactions, it should be discussed with your physician who will likely suggest adjusting dosage or changing the medication. As there are numerous types of analgesics available on the market, it is likely you will be successful in finding one which is effective. If you are not able to tolerate painkillers (a rare possibility), you can still use the mind to help control the pain. Your family physician may need to consult with a pain specialist for recommendations of appropriate medication. Few family physicians are trained in the management of chronic pain. This is not their fault: Most medical schools in Northern America do not teach how to treat chronic pain. In fact, our medical sources tell us that the very existence of chronic pain is frequently denied today.

Myth: Opioids cause serious withdrawal effects when you stop taking them. Many medications, not only the opioids, will have withdrawal effects when their use is terminated abruptly. For this reason most medications should be slowly decreased and not totally cut within one day. Opioids are not different from other medications and can be slowly reduced without causing excessive stress to the body. The dramatic accounts of withdrawal among street addicts seem to reflect an interaction between the feeling of sudden withdrawal from high dose usage and some characteristics of certain addictive personalities. Sudden medication withdrawal should usually be avoided. Clients do well to always discuss with their physician how to taper medication. Everybody should also know that insulin, antidepressants and blood pressure medications, to name only a few, can have serious withdrawal symptoms. However it is politically correct to use insulin and it is not politically correct to use opioids. Therefore withdrawal effects are often presented as something unique to opioids. Indeed, where they occur with the SSRI antidepressants, they are called "Discontinuation Syndrome" rather than "withdrawal symptoms."

Outside of its use as a marketing technique, the purpose of this nomenclatural distinction is unclear to us. Dr. Helen Hays, a leader in chronic pain management and a specialist in palliative care, with a private practice in Edmonton (Alberta, Canada) confirmed that her goal is to control the pain before it destroys life. She says she treats the pain until clients have zero pain and then slowly takes all the medication away. She also confirms the pain often then stays away. The goal is to reach the right balance with medication, heal your life, connect with your community and be happy. Then you can begin to reduce opioids totally or partly if you can, and pain may stay away.

Your family physician and your pain specialist will support you in your medication needs in this long road to recovery. You should not stop taking narcotics on your own, without the guidance of a physician, in the middle of a broken life. Other caregivers, such as physical therapists and psychologists, should also be there to support you in your odyssey for healing.

Myth: Treatment of chronic pain with opioids will cause addiction. Many users develop tolerance to many medications, however this myth is not true for the following reasons: tolerance and addiction are not the same, addiction is a disease preventing someone from functioning properly and forcing the person into compulsive use of a substance, even if that substance causes negative results. These destructive effects include damage to families, careers, and health in general. The addict continues to take the substance in spite of these effects. Addiction prevents one from functioning properly.

On the other hand, therapeutic use of opioids assists people with pain to function properly with positive results. It allows people to work, have a family and a good quality of life while addictions cause the opposite results. As Fishman explains, "the pain patient does better and the addicted patient does worse." Over a number of years,

Dr. Russell Portenoy studied almost twenty-five thousand cancer clients who had been on opioid therapy for many years. Of the entire group, only seven showed any signs of abuse.[10] Current fear of addiction pushes physicians to not prescribe opioids and also clients not to request them. The irony is that traditionally opioids were prescribed to everyone for any kinds of medical conditions and only recently have opioids been associated with addictions.[11] Medicine and pharmacology have been, so far, unable to present a safer and better substitute for the opioids. For this reason we expect opioids will remain in many homes.

Myth: Oxycontin ® is highly addictive. Oxycontin® has been and is still a target for criticism as a highly addictive opioid. Oxycontin® is a long-acting opioid preparation. It is not addictive when taken as prescribed. People with addiction issues use Oxycontin® illegally by buying it off the street or stealing it. Oxycontin® pills have a time release structure that allows the medication to be gradually absorbed when taken as prescribed. People with addictions usually crush the pill and snort or inject the resulting powder, causing the entire dose to be released at once. Unfortunately this use of Oxycontin® has received wide publication, and many people now believe they will develop an undesirable addiction in taking intact pills. Users should remember they must swallow the entire pills and do not take them in the same way as addicts do. They should also know they will likely get pain if they do not take their medication as prescribed. Pain is the reminder that medication is needed (and ideally, analgesic medication should be taken before pain becomes overwhelming). As long as analgesic medication is taken only as prescribed, addictive disorders are unlikely to result.

Myth: If people know I take opioids, I will be

assaulted by illegal users wanting to steal my pills, and my life will be at risk. The very small risk of this is often exaggerated. I have spoken with physicians and pain specialists, who had never been assaulted. Their houses had never been broken into by drug seekers. One physician reported that she leaves her car open because she does not want anyone to break her windows to access possible medication. However these people have never had problems associated with being known for prescribing opioids to their clients.

Myth: People taking opioids are terminally ill. Not true! These medications can be taken at any time in life, even in childhood. People who use opioids, may not feel that this practice is accepted by society and they may expect to receive negative judgment from the healthy. They do not always reveal the nature of their prescription. Have you ever thought the ones using therapeutic narcotics could be your mother or your sister or your spouse or the nice mother next door? It is impossible to know from the outside. Considering the negative social connotation of narcotic use and perception that only people waiting for imminent death use opioids, do you blame the non terminally ill person for not revealing the use of a narcotic?

Myth: A long term release opioid, when combined with alcohol, can be lethal. People have died because of this combination. Truth is you should always drink a moderate amount of alcohol, especially if you take medication. Alcohol changes the way medications are absorbed by the body. Unfortunately people wishing to die because of their pain, may use the combination of a large quantity of alcohol with an overdose of medication when they decide to commit suicide. Scientific data on the impact of alcohol on opioids are still a subject under research and it is misleading to use tragedies as a valuable source of objective data on the general use of alcohol and opioids. In spite of ongoing research, unwanted effects of various medications are still unknown, so when you take your analgesics you do well to pay attention to the way your body reacts. You will notice many benefits and you will learn to deal with the unwelcome effects. You should communicate the impact of your medications to your medical team.

Myth: There is somewhere a magic pill to remove chronic pain. Unfortunately there is no magic pill. Methods to manage pain can be learned and practiced. Medication can help. However magic pills do not exist. As you make peace with chronic pain, your body and your life are healed and the pain is transformed into something you accept.

Myth: You must suffer and no remedy is available. There are numerous ways to significantly decrease pain and feel better. Medication helps and there is an extraordinary number of painkillers. Strategies for relaxation and management of medical conditions exist. They can be combined with the traditional treatment by medication. Psychological factors alone rarely cause persistent pain but they can trigger or worsen pain and contribute to distress and disability. Several approaches exist to deal with these factors and help people develop a sense of mastery over pain. Psychological strategies for coping with pain work by helping control physiological responses that contribute to pain production.[12] The secret is to try different medications and different alternative approaches as well as to persist and bond with people until we obtain some relief. We believe one approach is not sufficient and all of them described in this book should be tried in order to achieve acceptable pain management. A good relationship with our caregivers will also assist the medications and alternative treatments to promote pain relief. After all, if we like our caregivers, we want them to succeed and in order for them to succeed, we are forced by our mind to heal.

Myth: Pain prevents us from being an active part of society. Not true! Pain may, however, transform our activities or redirect our energy. It may slow down our commitments to others. It may be a sign that we need to take better care of ourselves and follow a healthier lifestyle. As we will see at the end of this book, pain can bring positive outcomes to us and others. In some cases, pain can provide us isolated time to create very important works which benefit society. Two such individuals are Charles Darwin who produced the *Origin of Species* and Florence Nightingale who developed basic instructions for the development of health care.[13] Both are still extremely influential. Charles Darwin (1809-1882) was a British scientist, geologist, naturalist and writer who developed the concept of natural selection as the source of all forms of life. His theory involving a few common ancestors and constant change in the evolution of species influenced modern science and philosophy. Florence Nightingale (1820-1910) was a British nurse, hospital reformer, humanitarian and writer. Her methods reduced the mortality rate of the sick and she undertook reforms within the health care system. In 1860 she opened a school of nursing and made nursing a medical profession. Without the chronic pain experienced by Charles Darwin and Florence Nightingale, lives of others may not have been enhanced. These two authors transformed their personal pain into altruism to make the world a better place for everyone.

Myth: If opioids are taken for a long time, they

will stop working. This belief is called "the ceiling effect." Apparently this only applies to certain medications but not to morphine and other opioids.[14] The truth is that doses of non-opioid medication usually increase over time to obtain continuing effective results. Unfortunately people believe this also applies to the opioids. This myth causes physicians to not prescribe opioids and clients to not take high enough doses to recognize good results.

Myth: If you take opioids on a regular basis to decrease pain in everyday life, it will become impossible to reduce pain if you need surgery or are seriously injured. This implies that our body gets used to painkillers and that these ones will not work any more if our pain increases. The truth is that several analgesics are available and can be taken if unexpected accidents or emergencies occur. Daily doses of opioids can be increased or combined with other painkillers to reduce pain. Did you know that if your chronic pain specialist lives in the town where you go to hospital for surgery or any other emergencies, you can ask to have this physician at the hospital where you are treated for unexpected medical conditions? The hospital physician treating you may refuse to invite your pain specialist at the hospital, however nothing prevents you from asking to have your pain specialist at the hospital to advise the other therapists and physicians on how to treat your chronic and acute pain.

Myth: Muscle relaxants should be discontinued after a few weeks because muscles become unable to relax on their own. According to this belief, medications control the muscles becoming dependent on them. The muscles are believed to lose their ability to control muscle spasms because the medications did that for them. My experience is that muscle relaxants are not effective at controlling ongoing and permanent muscle spasms. Analgesics, massage, proper posture and a healthy lifestyle with a better response to stress are my main tools for managing muscle spasms. We do not feel muscle relaxants have a significant impact on our muscles and we did not feel that our bodies became dependent on them.

Fact: Pain is a controversial issue dividing physicians, therapists, clients, friends, families. Just what you need when you hurt! Some people, including clinicians and specialists, believe that pain is a psychosomatic matter and not a physical condition. The truth is that suffering is psychological, pain is psychological or physical, and sometimes both are true. Surprisingly we live in a society interested in studying the effect of the mind over the body rather than the effect of the body on the mind. Depression can be the result of a condition that is physical, psychological, financial, social or any condition that is not welcome.

Fact: It is possible to negotiate peace with pain; circumstances can also change its intensity. If we receive good quality medical care, support and compassion from our medical team and our significant ones, if we develop connections with a community, our pain decreases. If we are happy, pain also decreases and even may sometimes totally disappear. I learned this many years ago, before the car accident, when my body and mind wanted to make a baby. I had three ectopic pregnancies without any physical pain, although pain around the uterus and the Fallopian is the usual first sign of such a pregnancy. I was very happy to be pregnant; my mind as well as my body wanted the babies and made it impossible for pain to take over me. Environmental and personal circumstances, then, have an important impact on pain.

Happiness tends to relieve pain very dramatically. For this reason, one does well to learn to develop positive emotions and to be altruistic and happy. A miracle will occur, your pain will decrease; you will ensure your survival and you will maintain an active role in society. At the same time, you will know yourself much better because pain has the power to force you to look at your body and your life, to negotiate peace with the physical parts and the events that hurt, to accept them the way they are. In general struggle increases pain and peace decreases it.

Fact: Feelings of happiness help to heal the body. The septum near the hypothalamus is the area of the brain associated with the experience of happiness. When this system is activated by therapeutic opioids, it develops endorphins reducing pain.[15] When this system is activated by other means causing feelings of pleasure (such as listening to music or admiring some beauty), endorphins are also created. They are even developed by healing expectations and placebos. Medications can increase reactions in the brain but do not create them. A symbol, such as a flower or a photo, is often sufficient to cause emotions and impact on the brain. The key is to have a positive emotional database or bank account holding pleasant sounds, images and tastes associated with pleasure, and to be able to recall these emotions when you wish to feel better.

Fact: Pain can be measured. Pain is invisible just like happiness, love or sadness. However in spite of pain being a feeling, we know pain exists and we can estimate its intensity even if this is challenging. How do we assess pain? It is accepted that a malfunction of the body implies a certain amount of pain; for example if you can't bend your back or turn your head, it is believed this disability will cause some pain. A therapist or a person with chronic pain can feel, on injured areas, muscle spasms or trigger points which go along with pain.

Fact: Medications create well-being by reducing pain and improving quality of life; however medication should not be the only therapy used by persons experiencing chronic pain. It is good to combine physical and mental therapies with medication because a combination of various ways to deal with pain gives options and increases freedom. Reduction of pain and improved quality of life from medication make life more enjoyable, but do not ensure happiness.

Fact: Our medical specialists can transplant organs and treat an incredible amount of illnesses. However pain, the most widely spread medical issue, escapes treatment and some forms of pain, such as neuropathic (or nervous system) pain, are usually still impossible to treat properly.

This statement is true and can be seen as a medical failure in our modern world. Pain statistics increase at a rapid rate because more people recover now than ever from accidents and illnesses. We live in an aging population, and increased stress levels exist in our society. In spite of the need to find solutions, there are few medical authorities in the area of pain management, and pain does not stand high on the medical hierarchy interested primarily in spectacular research involving advanced technology. General practitioners are usually not trained in care for chronic pain clients. This occurs in a world which still suffers from untreated pain, when at the same time we are able to explore the planet Mars and are not ashamed to spend billions of dollars on this kind of research.

Fact: Pain tends to be treated as an illness and a medical condition. This is a mixed blessing. It is positive because it gives pain a medical status and, consequently, makes medications and disability programs more accessible. This also removes the fact that pain is emotional and medication is not the only solution because numbers of chronic pain sufferers increase in spite of the tons of Aspirin® consumed by Americans per year.[16]

Fact: Pain is undertreated. Too many perceptions still exist to allow people to receive medication removing pain. Many people still suffer because pain is so misunderstood. A few years ago Tracy Latimer, a 12 year-old severely disabled Saskatchewan (Canada) girl, was killed by her father using carbon monoxide. He was later sent to jail for murder and as a consequence forced to abandon the remainder of his family. It was claimed that Tracy "couldn't be treated with the usual analgesics because of the anticonvulsive medication she was on" and at least one pain specialist disagreed with this statement.[17] This death gave rise to numerous discussions on human rights and ethical issues. The debate should have began with a discussion about pain and the reasons why Tracy (and other North American children with chronic pain) did not and still do not get proper pain relief when medical treatments exist that can allow it.[18] Don't we know enough about pain to treat it properly?

Fact: It is easier in North America for teenagers to handle drugs in schools than for someone with chronic pain to receive pain relief. We recently attended in Edmonton a community party where one guest, a math teacher, explained to us how policemen and drug-sniffing dogs, came to the upper class high school where he worked: one student rolled a joint on his knees and passed it to another. The little police dog, a beagle if we remember well, pushed its nose against the teen until the police noticed it and only then interviewed the student. Apparently drugs and weapons, including guns and knives, were found in students' lockers. This is not an unusual occurrence. Most students in Northern American junior and senior high schools have at least been exposed to drugs and at least 5% take illegal drugs on a regular basis according to sources mentioned to me during conversations with my local city police. Real figures may even be higher. Recipes to make the most dangerous drugs from common ingredients found over the counter in drugstores are found on Internet. Teenagers take illegal drugs to deal with stress, emotions, family issues or to have the impression they perform better.

At the same party we heard the sad story of Bryan, a senior who had intractable serious chronic pain in his legs and who had no access to narcotics that could improve the quality of his life. While most medical doctors are not trained to treat chronic pain, they must also be very careful when prescribing narcotics for fear of sanction. As a consequence of scientifically unfounded negative attitudes, several physicians are regularly exposed to malpractice litigation by their clients even if they did receive proper training. We agree that our society has a "love-hate relationship" with legal and illegal drugs. It remains very upsetting to know that Canada spends "$2 billion a year putting drug offenders in jail while denying opiates to the hospitalized elderly, half of whom die in pain."[19]

Fact: The legalization and use of marijuana as a pain reliever are made difficult because the pharmaceutical companies can't obtain a patent for a plant and make revenues from it. Marijuana has been used for several thousands years because it offers almost immediate pain relief and it has anti-inflammatory and anti-spasmodic benefits. However it is still largely unavailable to the ones with chronic pain although legislation allows it in some countries such as Canada. It can grow very easily in gardens in North America. Smoking the leaves, even a very small quantity, is sufficient to increase sleep and appetite as well as to relieve pain among people with AIDS. Minimal effort is made to have marijuana available to them and other people. First of all, AIDS is not a politically correct disease. In addition, pharmaceutical companies control the availability of medications and marijuana will not be easily available until it can be administered widely as a puff or a pill. When it is available as a product to be purchased from a pharmacy and when it brings millions of dollars of revenues, it will then be available to people with chronic pain.

Fact: Physicians exert effects through their beliefs. This means that if they strongly prefer a therapy, this therapy can have a strong impact on the client. The relationship between physician and client is the therapeutic agent, not the technique which can be ineffective by itself. Suggestions from the physician can aid recovery by letting the client believe he or she will do better. These beliefs have been proven to be more effective than a placebo and reveal that "there is some aspect of the human psyche capable of shaping events in our world."[20] Several medical agents are effective alone, whatever a doctor's beliefs, but this indicates the importance of connecting with the right physician. Doctors' beliefs are usually influenced by marketing campaigns attached to a new pharmaceutical product. Some medication can work well as long as it is new and physicians believe it is effective. As soon as these beliefs become negative, the medication's effectiveness decreases.[21]

Fact: It is an unwise scientific practice to leave medical research in the hands of vested inter-

ests as has been done with medication research throughout the western world. Of course research must have a source of funding. However financial matters have a huge impact on the mind of researchers and if your mind is being influenced by financial matters, it is not objective. This means that research financed by pharmaceutical companies is well appreciated by users needing new medication, but this research may bring several results of interest to the sponsoring companies. Results indicating equally effective non-medication based treatments may go unattended. In the same area, free samples of new medication are essential to promote these products, but any products given at no cost to physicians will influence them when it is time for them to prescribe medication.

Fact: Chronic pain kills. Please do not allow yourself to ignore this fact. Cancer tumors grow much faster when pain is present.[22] Pain can destroy the nervous system and can cause a dysfunction of the immune system. Pain decreases resistance to stressors and causes depression. Pain or fear of it often leads to assisted or non-assisted suicide. All in all, pain, if not managed, can take away your life. You are far too precious to give away this life to pain! Please keep in mind there are people who care for you and wish to support you in your quest for peace with your pain even if they do not know how to help you.

Fact: Chronic pain is a disease by itself and not just a symptom of another problem. It has been observed that the brain of someone with chronic pain produces proteins uncommon in the brains of persons without pain. It is also obvious that opioids can prevent a healthy person from being able to concentrate when, on the other hand, they help people in pain to concentrate and to be alert. The impact of pain on the body is a new research field of study for scientists.

Fact: People experiencing chronic pain must develop endorphins to reduce pain. This can be accomplished with the use of medications, physical exercises, psychotherapy, mind power or spirituality. Simply enjoying life, through nature or the arts, has a positive impact on developing endorphins.[23] Connecting with people is another great way to boost endorphins. Some persons with arthritis are reported to have from 30% to 86% less endorphins than healthy people.[24] Development of endorphins is a survival necessity. However too many endorphins can cause additional pain and be bad for health, such as endorphins resulting from stress. Excessive exercise may produce an excess of endorphins in the body and an insufficient amount in the brain. This imbalance is dangerous.[25] The essential point here is about the importance of maintaining a good balance through activities producing endorphins.

Fact: You can develop a tolerance to a painkiller and doses will have to be increased. Tolerance is normal. Our body, under the leadership of the mind, develops tolerance to all types of stressors and to just about anything else presented to it. This is the reason why the body should be congratulated for its power of adaptability. We can develop tolerance to milk or spicy food, and if we take the same medication for a number of years, larger doses may need to be taken to produce the same effect. This can be avoided by using several analgesics at the same time, such as Neurontin® and Oxycontin®. If we mix two or more painkillers, a compound benefit will occur and increase results. Smaller doses can then be maintained for longer periods. New painkillers keep appearing on the market and if one becomes less effective, another one may replace it.

Your pain specialist is the best person to calculate doses and prescribe analgesics. There is no fixed "menu" because people differ in their responses to different medications. An analgesic good for someone may not be the best for you. Typically medication trials start with a small dose of one or two types of painkillers. It is best to start when you do not have to work and can rest. You report any side effects and your comfort level to your physician who knows which medications are compatible and will adjust doses accordingly. It may take a month or more before your "menu" is set. Ideally pain is reduced allowing you to remain alert and able to continue your normal activities.

Fact: Antidepressants can be used to decrease pain.
Antidepressants are used to reduce emotional pain and can be of assistance in increasing the quality of sleep and it is usual for comfort to improve during the day following a good night of sleep. Antidepressants alter the chemical transmitters of nerve impulses. This makes them useful in reducing emotional pain although there may be some unwanted "side effects." These last two words are marketing terms used to define effects we don't want since it is normal for a medication to make an effect. In addition, it is uncommon to suffer from chronic pain without suffering from depression, and antidepressant therapy helps manage mild depression by providing general feeling of well-being which is essential for healing. I noticed that tricyclic antidepressants are effective in reducing the constant burning pain which is extremely difficult to control. As a cautionary note, just as analgesics may obscure the identification of the source of the physical pain, so may antidepressants obscure the identification of the sources of emotional pain. This can interfere with psychotherapy.

Fact: Opioids change the perception of pain.

This means opioids do not cure pain even if they help to decrease pain and to increase quality of life as well as level of activities. This means they allow you to have a good night of sleep, to enjoy leisure activities, to socialize and of course to maintain a working position. Pain is still there but decreases enough for the body to function better. Morphine works by attaching itself to a receptor on the surface of a cell, causing the receptor to send a signal, into the cell, alleviating pain. In other words opioids block the transmission of pain signals. Although morphine is one of the oldest known analgesics, research is still needed to fully understand its pain reducing mechanism.

Fact: Side effects are not the same for people taking same or similar medication. Opioids are said to cause constipation while other painkillers can cause dry mouth, dizziness and/or drowsiness. Not everyone will experience any or all side effects to medications. Our experience is that side effects can usually be managed in the same manner as pain. Don't you feel that, if you can manage pain, you should be able to manage side effects from medication? Large glasses of water taken during the day, a diet rich in fruit and fibers, good quality of sleep, faith in your recovery and connecting with the right people at the right time and place, help remove many secondary effects. We cannot usually predict if side effects will occur until we actually use the medication. The printed information provided by pharmacists may be useful, but covers all known side effects; you will most likely not experience all of these secondary effects. Therefore medications prescribed to you by a trusted physician should be used on a trial basis before anticipating their side effects.

It is probably fair to say that any medication therapy will have a higher rate of success when it does not become one's sole preoccupation. Medications are only one method of treatment, and they cannot function well when other methods are ignored or used in disarray.

Fact: Fear magnifies pain. This concept is unique for everyone, however fear is almost certain to increase pain.[26] Of course it also has an impact on stress and can make it difficult to function properly. Psychological strategies to help cope with pain, such as deep breathing, will also help reduce fear. The key is to manage fear and disconnect it from physical pain. Having faith in one's potential to manage pain effectively decreases fear.

Fact: Pain treatments often fail because they are too complex and involve too many health professionals. Of course something too complex is bound to fail. Each therapist is responsible for one type of care or one part of the body. The client is usually the contact person for all these caregivers, and communications can be difficult and stressful, especially if the client has serious pain.

Fact: There is much about pain medicine which is still left to discover. Tylenol® is a very common analgesic. Medical science is knowledgeable about its function however it is not yet clear how it relieves pain and other symptoms.[27] It is known that Tylenol® reduces pain at the beginning of an episode but increases pain after a little while.[28] Despite Tylenol® being a household word, we remain largely ignorant of its precise mechanism of action. The same is true for the action of ASA or acetylsalicylic acid. We know in general how cocaine functions; however we still do not understand its molecular activity. In addition, we do not always know why combined medications work well. On the other hand, most clinical trials are performed on men and on Caucasians rather than Asians or Africans. These last two races appear to require smaller doses.[29] Much work is still needed as to exact dosing and absorption of medication by different metabolisms.

Fact: A growing number of North Americans take prescription medications not only to reduce occasional pain but also to increase performance. These products include stimulants, antidepressants, tranquilizers and other pills acting as mind enhancers. Clients who seek "cosmetic neurology" want to access medications when they are generally healthy. An estimated 20% to 25% of Canadians take advantage of these psychotropic medications according to a 2005 study published by Lianne George in *Maclean's*. The fact is these people sometimes purchase mind lifting medication from legitimate users if they cannot obtain prescriptions from their regular physicians. It is true certain medications can enhance or reduce mental function. This creates ethical issues faced by physicians and clients. Long term effects of neurochemicals are generally unknown and incompletely documented.

Fact: The brain of a person living with chronic pain is different from a healthy person's brain. Opioids administered to people with chronic pain allows them to function better. However the same doses may prevent a person not in pain from functioning by causing strong side effects such as drowsiness. There is still much to investigate and understand in this area. Clinical trials typically do not include the healthy controls. This makes comparisons more difficult. Pain is a feeling but it often indicates a pathological condition, such as injured soft tissues. Many conditions can cause pain and one does well to make one's own decisions to facilitate one's own recovery. You are your own judge and will do well to try all therapies reasonable to you. You should retain the therapies you find the most helpful. This is not easy because there is no official therapy to recommend. Please remember you are on an odyssey with specific needs and your quest for healing is your own.

Fact: We do not have to know why treatments work before using them. If medications are safe and do not cause unpleasant side effects, they can be taken if they are successful in decreasing pain and increasing quality of life. General anesthesia would not have spread beyond ether if doctors insisted on knowing with precision how medications work.[30] Anti-inflammatories have long been used for pain relief before scientists discovered exactly how they worked. In fact, Aspirin® 's effects are still only partly understood. The use of antibiotics would have been significantly delayed if scientists had needed to know how penicillin worked before using it.[31] It is better to first ask the question "Does it work?" before asking "How does it work?" After all, if it does not work, who cares how it doesn't work?

Fact: Opium meaning "juice" in Greek is a poppy extract and has been used for several thousands of years to reduce pain. In the *Odyssey* about 1000 B.C. Ulysses and his companions are exposed to potions extracted from a plant and bringing forgetfulness; it is believed these drinks contained opium. One of the first scientifically documented formulations was created in the 16th century by a chemist named Paracelsus who mixed opium with alcohol and possible other ingredients such as frog sperm and cinnamon. This concoction was called "laudanum."[32] Morphine, opium's most potent metabolite, was first extracted from the plant in 1803 by a German scientist. Its use expanded when doctors learned how to inject it into the bloodstream. In the later part of the 19th century opium was openly available in stores in the US. However in the early 1900s the US started to restrict use of opioids and in 1914 the Harrison Act, the first American law restricting the use of certain medications, was passed.

Those three were quick to find the Lotus-Eaters,
who did not think of slaughtering my men:
in fact, they shared their lotus food with them.
Those three who feasted on the honey-sweet,
enticing lotus fruit had not the least
desire to bring back word or soon return
at all: they wanted only to stay there,
to feed upon that food and disremember
their homeward path. I had to force them back,
in tears, to their own ships; there, they were dragged beneath
the rowing benches and bound fast. And I had all my other firm companions
embark with speed upon our rapid ships,
that no one –tasting lotus- might forget
his homeward way.

Ulysses about his companions coming back from the Trojan wars, *Odyssey*, 1990, original book IX, 91-119, written around 800 B.C. We suggest this lotus fruit refers to poppy seeds or opium.

In 1875 chemists added two acetyl groups to morphine and created the first semisynthetic derivative which was later named heroin. Twenty years later the Bayer Company gave this substance the trade name "heroisch" for its strong and heroic qualities. Heroin was born and used to treat coughs and diarrhea. It was marketed as a non-addictive alternative to morphine. Later alterations to opium brought numerous other analgesic preparations, including codeine (a more natural version which theorically does not cross the blood-brain barrier), meperidine (now known as

Demerol®) which in 1939 became the first synthetic opioid, methadone (another synthetic version developed in Germany during World War II), hydromorphone (now known as Dilaudid®) which is 10 times stronger than morphine and fentanyl now administered in patch form as it can be absorbed through the skin.

At the beginning of the 20th century Canada restricted the use of opioids, however the early 1960s saw Canada as the first western jurisdiction to authorize methadone use to treat opiate addiction. At the beginning of the 21st century, several pain authorities support the therapeutic use of long term opioids to reduce chronic pain, even if the use remains controversial in public opinion. Opioids have been used for several thousands of years, and it is probably safe to assert that they will be used many decades to come.

Fact: The gold standard of pain analgesic in terms of medication is still the opiates, which are made from herbs, despite the advances of biotechnology and chemical engineering. Throughout the ages opium has been used to treat such things as gallbladder pain, kidney stones, headaches, asthma, insomnia and toothaches. It was commonly used on battlefields during the last two centuries to treat wounded soldiers. Pharmaceutical manufacturers have so far been unable to produce other alternative analgesic medications which are more efficient than opioids, in spite of the millions of dollars spent on constant research and in spite of modern knowledge and almost unlimited means of research.[33]

Fact: There is irony in opiate phobia (fear of opiates). Heroin initial use was to treat coughs, and ironically codeine – an opiate – is still considered an excellent cough medication. It is available in most households. Most people do not know the connection between heroin and the pretty red syrup in the family refrigerator. When coca was introduced to Europe from South America around 1859, it was extracted into medicinal wine and twenty years later, John Pemberton, a Georgia chemist, used the plant to create the medicinal drink he named Coca-Cola. In 1906 coca was replaced by caffeine in this same drink. Then, in 1860 a German scientist mixed coca leaves with water and other solvents to produce pure cocaine. This innovative medicinal product was used to energize and fight depression. The neurologist and psychologist Sigmund Freud used it to treat psychological disorders and to invent local anesthesia, a monumental contribution in the history of medicine.[34]

Most people ironically do not understand the connection between Coca-Cola, cocaine and a powerful agent allowing surgery. Also relatively unknown is the direct link between cocaine and Novocain, and other anesthetics with names ending in -"cain" which produce numbing effect without affecting mood. Just last week we overheard a pharmacist explaining, to a mother and her child, that one of these preparations, ending in -"cain", was a marvelous product to stop mosquito bite pain and sunburn pain on a child's skin!

Fact: People on opioid therapy are dependent. However in reality their physical needs are far away from what is referred to as addiction by medical professionals and governments. "Addiction is a psychological condition that compels a person to satisfy that need, and keep satisfying it, no matter what."[35] "Dependence is a physical state that occurs when the lack of a drug causes the body to have a reaction."[36] Addiction and dependence are very different. Addiction has a large psychological component.

Dependence, if medication is abruptly discontinued, leads to severe physical issues such as sweating, racing heart and nausea. People develop tolerance and dependence to most things, including food, medications and noise. Apparently addiction to gambling is the most common addiction.

Many people are dependent on tea, coffee or other drinks and do not feel badly at all about their dependence, it in fact seems to be normal. We should also remember that when opioid medication is stopped, withdrawal symptoms do not kill. However in cases of other medications, such as insulin and all the ones used for hypertension, withdrawal can kill. After all, dependence on opioid therapy does not seem so terrible when taken into a larger context.

Fact: A placebo can be a very effective way to modify or reduce pain. Placebos include things such as magic, faith, suggestions from an authority, expectation to heal and confidence in a health care provider. In various large studies, anywhere from one-quarter to three-quarters of clients react well to placebos.[37] There is little agreement on the number of people reacting well to placebos.[38] Why are these positive results from placebos occurring? Maybe the medical condition is best treated with time. Possibly clients react well because they trust the treatment or the doctor. It is well known that positive beliefs, on which placebos and medications are based, have a large impact on the body. Placebos may help reduce anxiety and most placebos reflect the natural interaction between the mind and the body.[39] Much remains unknown, such as when the analgesic effect will occur, how long it will last and what kinds of persons can the most benefit from placebos.

In an Hippocratic text entitled *Epidemics* we read that "Nature, without instruction or knowledge, does what is necessary." Placebos or recovery from illness without any intervention were already known by ancient Greeks. The word "physician" is derived from the Greek "physis" meaning "nature" and nature is "the core of healing's secret."[40] Nuland also believed that "the magic that has always been intertwined with medicine is no less a part of healing today than it has ever been – it simply comes in a different costume... the red body paint and extravagant headdress of the primitive healer have been replaced with the white coat... even today, magic is often part of the cure, and in some situations it is the entire cure."[41] Chrome plated equipment was also added to the white coat. Placebos are as old as the world and they always have been a component of health care. In the 5th century B.C., Hippocrates knew that "Some patients, though conscious that their condition is perilous, recover their health simply through their contentment with the goodness of the physician"[42] and this belief is still accepted by several physicians.[43] It is now believed that, if a placebo does not reduce the pain level, the simulated medication is not part of the user's culture and this could be the reason for the lack of positive outcomes. It could also be that the physician and the client are not effectively and efficiently connecting. Placebos and many other medications are based on hope, and the results will not be reached if faith is not there.[44] You should also be aware that it is illegal and unethical to give a placebo without the user's permission. In a clinical trial using placebos, people do not always know when a placebo is used, but they must sign consent for the trial and should be told that placebos will be used in this project. Of course a physician or any other therapists giving a placebo to a client, without telling the client, will also destroy trust in the relationship with this person.

Fact: Opioids for chronic pain do not cause eupho-

ria. This medication is time-released or long-acting, and taken into the body as pills or patches. It is not injected and goes slowly into the bloodstream. It does not speed to the brain. You do not see an immediate relief. It takes a few days for the medication to decrease the pain level and even when you are used to it, you should count at least 30 min for chronic pain to decrease after ingesting a pill. Taking opioids is little different than taking Tylenol® or Aspirin®. My personal experience is that opiates are more effective at decreasing moderate and severe pain that did not responded to other analgesics.

Fact: Opioids do not completely remove the pain. Pain will be present but less severe. Opioids provide "extra endorphins" to the body. Doses are calculated to ensure the user functions well without appearing medicated, confused or dozed. Usually physicians prescribe a small dose and gradually increase it to an effective and safe level. The goal is to reduce your suffering and allow you to improve your function at work, in the family and community. The user will be able to enjoy life but will also continue to have an acceptable level of pain and should add to the chronic pain management plan other approaches, such as psychotherapy. If you have some pain, if you are happy and if you function well, you may not need opioids. If not, you do well to consider whether this is a solution for you. You should always discuss with your physician if you feel your pain is not adequately controlled. Opioids eliminate some chronic pain but may not affect other pains. They may allow you to feel as close to normal as possible. They will not heal your life but can greatly facilitate your recovery. They are important components of your therapy and will help you sign a peace treaty with pain. If someone uses opioids for pain, this person will still feel acute pain (such as burning a finger), as a non-opioid user. Yes, narcotics allow you to feel even mosquito bites while pain from muscle spasms will slowly decrease.

Fact: Opioids have a terrible social association. Unfortunately this is true. Many people, perhaps including many of your loved ones such as spouse, children and/ or parents, may believe you are a drug addict (or on the way to becoming one) if they know you manage your pain with opioids. Just when you need support from them, they may judge you in a negative way. This can be very difficult especially when one of your goals is to bond with people in your quest for recovery. Hopefully education on an on-going basis about your opioid medication will reduce negative reactions. You may want to organize a meeting with your physician and your significant ones, as a part of this educational process. Most physicians will agree to speak to your family and discuss their concerns so long as you are in agreement. Medication may bring you new friends. If support does not come from your family, you may look for support somewhere else among your friends and your community. Please do not forget this is your pain, and it is your choice to deal with it according to what **you** wish to do. No one has the right to judge you and no one should be critical of the way you choose to deal with your pain.

Fact: The brain produces a natural opiate that helps to reduce pain. The brain's natural morphine started to be recognized in the early 1970s when Avram Goldstein at Stanford University devised a chemical test to locate opiate-like molecules. He searched for binding sites or receptor cells designed to catch molecules working like morphine. Tests were performed by grinding animal brains and filtering the mixture through radioactive chemicals which attached to the specific receptors. In 1973

Solomon Synder from Johns Hopkins University found opiate receptors in the brain cells of mice. The brain's natural opiates were located three years later by Scottish scientists. They labelled them "enkephalin" (Greek word meaning "from the head"). American scientists have named similar opioids "endorphins," a term that combines the words "endogenous" (meaning "produced in the body") with "morphine." Another form of natural opioids were discovered and named "dynorphins." These three terms for the natural opioids are the results of a race between American and European scientists. The term "endorphins" (invented by the Americans) eventually overtook the other words.[45]

Fact: Natural opioid receptors are found all over our bodies in intestines, the stomach, glands, central nervous system and the brain. These seem to be involved in several bodily functions and suppress the body's production of chemicals associated with damaged tissue. Exercise, sexual activity and the need to survive an immediate physical trauma increase the endorphin levels. These levels also increase significantly among pregnant women during labor.[46]

Fact: We still do not know how the mind controls specific natural chemicals and interacts with the rest of the body. Some placebo responses may involve endorphins. Blocking endorphins with naloxone can, in certain cases, block the pain relief resulting from placebos. It is believed there is a neurochemical basis to the mind. In a placebo, faith or belief somehow turns on the neurochemicals including the endorphins. We do not know the details of this action.[47] Chronic pain is an extremely complex field full of unknown components.

Fact: A medication including two ingredients such as a narcotic and a regular analgesic is not

recommended by doctors even if it has less narcotic than a common 100% opioid. These medications are not recommended for chronic pain to be taken for a long period of time because the analgesic component can have an impact on the liver and kidneys. Quite often medication must be increased and this means the rising level of (for example) acetaminophen may place individuals at risk for liver damage. It is impossible to increase one ingredient without increasing the other when both are in the same tablet. Taking two different tablets instead of one that combines the two ingredients is desirable because it allows independent adjustments of the amounts of each component.

Fact: There are numerous types of opioids, and if one does not work, it is possible to change and try another one. Many people are fortunate to have success with the first medication they use. Happily there is a variety of opioids available because variation in individual responsiveness is common. The most frequently prescribed opioids include the following:

- Short acting: Actiq® (fentanyl), Darvon® (propoxyphene), Demerol® (meperidine), Dilaudid® (hydromorphone), MSIR® (morphine), Percocet® (oxycodone and acetaminophen), Roxicodone® (oxycodone), Tylenol® 3 and 4 (codeine and acetaminophen), Vicodin® (hydrocodone and acetaminophen)

- Long-acting or delayed action (useful in chronic situations): Duragesic® (fentanyl transderm), Dolophine® (methadone), MS Contin® (morphine, slow release), Oramorph SR® (morphine, slow release) and Oxycontin® (oxycodone).

The brand name is given first and the generic name

follows in parentheses. We know people who have said they would never take opioids …. while they were taking Tylenol© 3!

Fact: Marijuana is a medication of benefit to several people with chronic pain. Marijuana is a plant that is increasingly used in therapy to decrease pain. The plant holds 60 cannabinoids, including the Delta-9 THC that appears to be the major active ingredient of interest to us. The plants currently grown are 700% more powerful than the ones cultivated in the 1970s. Marijuana is inexpensive and rarely leads to dependency. Tolerance to cannabis is slow when compared with other medications; in fact, reverse tolerance has been commonly reported. However smoking is not a healthy way to obtain its therapeutical benefits. Smoking makes it more difficult to quantify doses. In addition, smoke is toxic. A spray has been developed to facilitate use of marijuana. The medication can be also mixed with food or hidden in a drink, but doses in food are also more difficult to calculate. Because research is ongoing, but still very limited, the unwanted effects of marijuana are better known than its benefits. Marijuana has been illegal for a long time in North America and for this reason much is still controversial. Several physicians are not comfortable with prescribing it because of myths attached to narcotics used as a medication and because of their lack of training with the use of opioids. Marijuana can produce euphoria, increase heart beat and distort time and space. It metabolizes in lungs and liver, and it has important effects on the reproductive system, including suppression of ovulation for women. However the benefits include increased appetite and decreased pain. Marijuana is believed to be of use to treat people with HIV/AID, multiple sclerosis, spinal cord injuries, seizures and muscle spasms. Its anti-inflammatory and anti-spasmodic benefits reduce the need to take several medications usually necessary in complex medical conditions. In addition marijuana treats depression and improves effectiveness of other medications. We should note that politicians and judges, not physicians, make final decisions on the legal use of marijuana. This seems a questionable practice.

Fact: It may be as important to take painkillers around the clock (even when there is no pain) as it is with other medications such as antidepressants. Many medications are long-acting and it is normal for their effects to continue when you believe you have no pain and no longer need them. If we have no pain, it can be the result of painkillers, not that our body has no pain. It is generally much easier to treat chronic pain with a regular program rather than to manage repeated crises. The goal of a regular program of medication used around the clock is to keep the pain under control and help attain our goal of an improved quality of life.

Fact: It is good to talk about your pain and your medication with people you trust. In addition to sharing your concerns with your physician, you may also release tension by discussing your concerns with significant and trusted people. It is important to find the right audience and the right way to express yourself. It is wise to not dramatize with children and older people who may tend to needlessly worry. One does well to keep in mind that some medications (i.e. opioids) continue to have a bad reputation. It is best to take medication in private and to exercise discretion in making known our use of analgesics. Privacy obviates the need to justify and explain to others, ensures safety and helps avoid gossip. It is a characteristic of human beings, sometimes endearing but more often irritating, that no amount of evidence suffices as proof to someone who wishes to remain unconvinced. When my children were young, they called my medications "vitamins." They understood that no one was allowed to touch them. They had their vitamins and I had mine. Now they are in late childhood, they know my "vitamins" are medications and they plan to one day invent one that will remove pain for ever. Meanwhile they understand that pain is part of life and that it is just more salient for some people. Charles Sherrington said that if the central nervous system only had one neuron over and above that needed to fulfill biological functions, that one neuron would mediate the perception of pain. It is then not outstanding to consider pain as attached to life.

In deciding to go public about my pain, I discovered that it is possible to derive some benefit from it. I believe my experiences may broaden knowledge about pain control and management. Our pain will not be a waste, and something good will be born from it. Our stories of personal battles with pain bring meaning, and become part of the important fight to improve health and medical care.

THE IRONY OF MEDICATION

Medication can only provide the best results within the context of an effective client/doctor relationship. Trust is essential to this relationship and to the pain management plan. If the client has no faith in the physician, he or she may decide to reduce dose or not comply with the prescribed regimen, especially where pesky side effects are present. It is well known that in a poor relationship medication does not produce the results one would predict from the research literature. Therefore bonding or connecting with a therapist is an ongoing and essential process that, when it succeeds, ensures faster physical improvement with smaller amounts of required medication and fewer secondary effects. At times medication can even be eliminated following an extended period of treatment.

THIS MAGICAL WORD CALLED BOTOX®

In the modern day press, Botox® seems to be the solution. It is also becoming a common word in the pain management world. Internet sites presenting the virtues of Botox®, in nearly every language, are increasing and the word appears on numerous advertisements in magazines and brochures. Botox® injections are one of the newest trends in pain management. Both professionals and businesses profit financially, so Botox® will continue to be marketed as a miracle solution surpassing many other products in its results.

What is Botox®? What is the publicity about Botox® not telling us? Ads do not say Botox® is one of the few most powerful natural poisons identified so far. One gram of this toxin could easily kill approximately 1.5 millions people.

Botox® is the common name for Botulinum Toxin A which is a protein structure. This potent biological toxin is transformed by simple dilution into a therapeutic agent treating a large variety of disorders characterized by muscle hyperactivity. Although Botox® is derived from the botulinum organism, this organism itself is never injected. The solution that is injected is the neurotoxin produced by the botulinum bacteria.

Working with Botulinum Toxin A as a therapeutic agent for treating human disease began in the late 1960s. The rights to a type of Botulinum Toxin A, commercialized under the trade name Botox® , were acquired in 1989 by Allergan and in December of that same year, the product was approved for use in the treatment of strabismus. Continuing development of this poison into a therapeutic agent still involves clinical trials attached to neurological disorders to allow better pain management for present and future generations.

Botox® is also being used extensively by dermatologists and plastic surgeons to reduce the appearance of wrinkles and soften facial lines. It is said to improve the quality of life of people with muscle spasms, headaches and neck pain, and to solve problems related to eyes, temporomandibular joint (TMJ) disorder, and to treat juvenile cerebral palsy. Nonetheless, the use of Botox® as a therapeutic agent is still very experimental and a few major Canadian universities, including the University of Alberta (Edmonton) and the University of Toronto, are conducting research on use of Botox® to treat pain and problems connected to it. This research involves injecting Botox® in the hope Botox® will become a standard agent to treat chronic pain.

Botox® is an example of the commercialization of pharmacotherapeutics. Potential huge revenues provide strong motivation for research, notwithstanding that most medical specialists are genuinely wishing to treat pain. Botox® may become the number one product for chronic pain treatment if research continues and is able to show positive results.

Botox® is not an easy substance to inject. A tiny syringe is used for multiple injection sites of medication into the muscle to be treated. The needle is usually connected to a wire attached to an electromyography (EMG) unit which records the activity of the muscle. The needle placement is verified by electrical signals indicated by the machine. When signals indicate the correct placement of the needle, the medication is injected.

MY TRIAL WITH BOTOX®

Four years ago, I participated in a long-term clinical trial at the University of Alberta. The goal was to study the impact of Botox® on TMJ disorder and related fascial cervical pain, which included muscle spasms and headaches. TMJ disorder also causes eating and speaking difficulties due to the limits it places on jaw mobility. It was hoped that Botox® injected into the area surrounding the temporomandibular joint, in the jaw and on the hairline would help alleviate pain, develop the bite force and improve the size of the mouth opening. My trial was blind, meaning the specialist and I did not know whether I received a Botox® or a placebo injection.

I found this trial very exciting because of the hopes and promises that have come to be associated with Botox®. I hoped a treatment that could assist many other people in pain would come from my own involvement. The procedure was fairly painful and I managed to practice breathing techniques during the 10 minutes or so of the 12 injections per treatment. Breathing relaxed the muscle and decreased the pain. I heard the sound of a noise similar to what I thought would be the sound of a running tap in my head. This was the result of the magnified noise of the solution being injected when the injections were in the area of the ears. No one warned me about this very uncomfortable noise, increasing the physical pain from the injections. To me, it was as if I was hearing the pain in addition to experiencing it physically.

My relationship with the specialist conducting the research was excellent and the nature of our relation was the primary reason I remained in the trial after realizing Botox® was not having a major impact on my pain. We managed to communicate although it was difficult to speak with the needle and the large amount of wiring. I do not know what the results from the clinical trial were and did not notice any decrease in my level of pain. No miracle occurred! I started the trial in pain and I left it in pain. The clinical trial did help me to practice breathing and develop better silent communication with physicians.

A CERTAIN HOPE ...

Botox® is not a cure, but for some it offers hope of a few months relief from pain and spasm. It is a long-acting neuromuscular blocking agent which causes local and temporary muscle paralysis by blocking the transmission of nerve impulses. It affects the muscle only where it is injected. At a normal neuromuscular junction, a nerve impulse triggers the release of acetylcholine, which causes the muscle to contract. The use of Botox® can be effective in blocking the release of acetylcholine at the neuromuscular junction and this prevents muscle contraction. This denervation takes 24-72 hours to occur after the injections and usually lasts from 3 to 6 months.

...WITH MAJOR CHALLENGES

Clinical use of Botox® presents several challenges. It is difficult to locate the exact muscles requiring treatment and to locate sites to inject. EMG equipment or a TENS unit can be used to localize the surface motor point over the muscle. However not every clinician is trained to use this equipment. Muscle contraction reduction often results in a lower muscle tone and muscle weakness. Repeated injections may be needed because recovery occurs when new nerve sprouts develop and establish new neuromuscular junctions. Some people may develop a tolerance to Botox® requiring increasingly larger doses of Botox®.

Correct doses are not formally established. A few sessions may be necessary to establish the correct one. Similar amounts do not always produce the same effect on the same muscle and on the same person. In the treatment of migraines, the optimal dose of Botox® is unknown and the most effective sites to be injected are still subject to debate. A fifteen minute injection session can be expensive (a few hundred dollars) and injections into damaged muscles are painful even to those with high thresholds to pain. Here is an essential point. If you wish to try Botox® to reduce chronic pain, please find a reassuring experienced specialist who communicates well because, as you remember, fear magnifies pain!

THE TRUTH ABOUT CLINICAL TRIALS

Clinical trials are experiments on human beings. They provide treatments on the cutting edge of research and give hope for an improved life, however they remain experiments. I was involved with use of Botox® to decrease symptoms of TMJ disorder with no guarantee about the results and I was not made aware of any benefits for myself and for others. There was pain that accompanied the injections and a few years later, the results are still unknown to me. Several participants stopped participating because of increase in their levels of pain, and others left Edmonton. Additional trials were required to be conducted to collect larger samples. At the time I assessed the adverse effects by researching Botox® and through discussion with one of the specialists conducting the trial. I accepted that I would not change my current medication at the time because the introduction of any new medication could affect the results from Botox®. My physicians agreed not to alter the amounts of my medication as well. If pain from my original injuries increased at the time or if pain increased because of the trial, I agreed not to increase my medication and I was instructed to use Tylenol®.

The University gave me large containers of Tylenol® without charge and I was asked to record the number of Tylenol® used to manage pain from the injections or from my medical condition. Parking was also provided. I decided to join the trial because I felt I could trust the specialist, conducting the testing on me, who agreed to be available at any time as a contact person during the study. We had many things to discuss outside the trial. He also did not use a visual EMG computer because it would force him to look away from me and directly at the screen just prior to the injection. Instead, he used a sound signal to ensure the needle was at the correct site. This allowed him to focus on me during the injection. I was also interested in finding a way to decrease my TMJ pain and being involved in medical research. My personal information would not be made available, however this was not at all a concern to me.

Many things should be considered if you decide to become involved in a clinical trial. There are questions and concerns that need to be addressed before agreeing to participate in a trial. Before giving your consent, the side effects, time involvement, procedures, benefits should be assessed. Access to your private information and, in general, your level of comfort with the trial should also be addressed. We should keep in mind that a trial is not a cure, and many do not bring free relief to pain. Many medications used during trials are not covered by health insurance plans. However trials do provide you with new information and access to specialists you might otherwise not have. It felt good to know we helped future persons with chronic pain by facilitating research. After all, something good should come from our pain.

An important part of the decision to be involved in any clinical trials is the contract you will need to sign. You are protected by the Nuremberg code of 1946 stating in the opening line that "The voluntary consent of the human subject is absolutely essential."[48] Before providing consent, you must be informed of benefits and risks related to the trial. Read the agreement thoroughly and ask questions you may have. The contract from the University had a provision for me to withdraw at any time, provided free medical care for any research-related injuries, and gave me the right to ask questions regarding the study.

Signing a written contract is essential. You should review it and ask any questions you may have before signing. You need to obtain a copy of this contract. Standard agreements usually include an introduction, your rights as a study participant, the purpose of the study with any experimental medication, the subject selection explaining what the selection criteria are, the procedure (explanation of all tests and procedures participants will undergo), risks and discomforts including side effects or potential complications, known benefits, alternatives if you choose not to participate, participation and withdrawal clause, cost and payment or compensation you may expect; a statement about injuries explaining who will pay for your medical care to treat research-related injuries and a note about confidentiality stating how researchers will ensure your personal information will be kept private. Not all consent documents include these clauses, so you need to question these areas if they are not included in your agreement.[49]

CHILDREN AND TRIALS

The number of clinical trials on children has grown dramatically since 1997. Regulations governing research involving children are rigid and studies approved for adults are illegal on children. Agreements must be signed by parents or guardians for participants under 18. Children have a right to equal access to advances in medicine and clinical trials allow better dosing of medication. Children also experience chronic pain. However medication can give them side effects that adults do not experience. Medications may cause them problems at one age (such as Aspirin®) and be safe at another age. Currently the American Food and Drug Administration encourages pharmaceutical manufacturers to conduct research with children and this will increase the number of clinical trials using children despite ethical reasons protecting children from the risks of research.[50]

In conclusion, at any ages you have options when you

use medication; your choice should be discussed with your medical team. Research on pharmaceutical products is ongoing. You should not hesitate to try new medication found on the market. Please do not judge a medication is not good for you without trying it and considering its secondary effects. One of the best rules is not to be afraid to combine and change medications when new products are available.

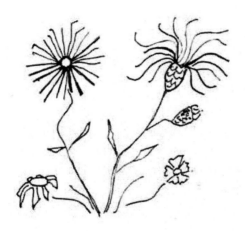

Chapter 3

PHYSICAL THERAPY

Physical therapy greatly helps to reduce mental suffering by establishing a physical contact with a therapist. Touching is one effective way to decrease pain. It is effective for trigger points, spasms, or any place where there is tension in the body. It is effective at any age: babies love to be picked up and rubbed; the dying also feel better when they are held. It is then not surprising that many who have chronic pain find physical therapies useful.

Sometimes the simple presence of a loved one can reduce chronic pain. If touching is added, pain may decrease even more. However you should keep in mind that touching injuries may well increase the pain before decreasing it. Of course I find this type of pain coming from caring hands easier to take than pain coming from wounds deep in the body; it is easier to remove suffering from pain when you are with a caregiver than when you are alone. For relief to happen in a professional setting, the client must establish a good relation with the caregiver. The nature of the relationship is as important as any physical therapy used by the caregiver.

Physical treatments cover several therapies but none of them works unless the one in pain is determined to do a share of work in managing pain. Here we suggest to be at peace with pain if you wish to benefit the most from physical therapy. It should be remembered that our bodies manufacture their own painkillers and routinely heal themselves. Increased by exercise and good nutrition, these painkilling agents include the endorphins, serotonin, and substance P. It is essential to believe these substances found in the nervous system will help you to decrease pain. Faith and hope create miracles in the world of chronic pain.

YOUR CHOICE

Physical therapies are important because our choice of food, our movement and exercise (or lack of it) are sources of healing or sources of pain. The good news is: we have the power, if we want, to follow physical therapies, get rid of factors harming us, and heal. Many of us hate to work in a gym and to calculate food groups; however it is a different story to be touched by strong and caring hands or go for a brisk walk in nature. Physical therapy becomes much easier to take when it comes in a form with which we are comfortable.

SOURCES OF PHYSICAL PAIN

Muscles may develop spasms with stress, or after an accident, or with poor posture, bad working positions, or repetitive movement. Muscles with spasms may become weak and tense up easily on an ongoing basis; painful spots called "trigger points" may develop as a consequence. Muscles found in the head, the neck and in the back are especially sensitive to stress. Shooting pain may also develop in the chest and is often mistaken for heart trouble. When muscle tightness persists, muscles are less able to work. Neck pain is common, and in many cases, it comes from injured muscles (for example as the result of a whiplash injury).

We know how muscle spasms feel. But what really happens when muscles spasm? A healthy muscle contracts when in use and relaxes when effort is finished. Muscles tense from stress and injury may go into spasms, sometimes because they are unable to relax any more, and sometimes because they protect an injured area by preventing it from working. Spasms are reflex reactions that are not consciously controlled.[1] Tension grows quickly in stiff muscles; blood is unable to circulate to nourish the muscle. Some tissues will degenerate and form little nodules called "trigger points" or "muscle knots." Pain can also manifest away from these points or knots. Of course the vicious circle is complete: Untreated trigger points continue to cause pain which increases tension of the muscle; this growing tension forces the muscle to contract more and creates additional trigger points …. And pain.

The TMJ (tempomandibular joint) can be an important location for this unfortunate circle. In TMJ pain syndrome, jaws are unbalanced and joints are out of alignment; muscles are consequently stressed especially as they keep working. Imbalance and stress cause muscle spasms and trigger points in the head, which are added to the long list of miseries found in the TMJ syndrome: blurred vision, headaches, earaches, pain in the neck, clicking sound when the mouth opens or closes, dizziness, ringing in the ears (tinnitus) and the like.

Physical treatments having a direct impact on muscles and soft tissues, are useful in managing muscle pain. One main goal of physical therapy is to release muscle spasms and heal the trigger points that so often cause pain.

MASSAGE AS A BENEFICIAL THERAPY

Worldwide, massage is the most common physical treatment. It is also one of the oldest therapies. In addition, massage is beneficial to the person giving it because it reduces depression, anxiety and pain among massage givers.[2] As a matter of fact, this is true: when I give a massage to one of my daughters suffering from a child illness, I totally block my own pain for as long as I focus on my child. Massage is often very painful for the one receiving it; this pain heals the body by removing toxins and bringing other benefits. Here in the western world, we are very distant from the idea of receiving massages for the pleasure of being touched in order to relax. We are in the middle of a pain management technique, often misunderstood because it does not belong to our traditional western medical system.

> The desire to touch and be touched is one of our most instinctive needs. The sense of touch is the first to develop in the embryo, and babies thrive on close physical contact with their mothers. The caring, loving touch of another is fundamental to the development of a healthy human being.
>
> Airey, *Healing Hands*, 2003, p.6.

Benefits from massages

Please don't let others' comments about how "lucky" you are to relax with massages, give you the impression that massages are a luxury. Therapeutic massage (in contrast to massage for relaxation enjoyed by the painless clients) can be important in a pain management plan for the mind and the body. According to my physical therapists, massage relaxes the mind, removes body toxins by draining them through the lymph system into the lymph nodes for purification; it increases endorphins, it calms down trigger points and spasms, relaxes muscles, increases blood circulation in injured areas, relieves stiffness and muscle knots, reduces the amount of stress hormones produced by the body, eases sleep, and has a significant impact on the nervous system. Massage blocks pain impulses from traveling up to the brain and apparently depletes substance P, a neurotransmitter involved in communicating the pain sensation.[3] Chronic pain signals travel on C-polymodal nerves at about 3 miles per hour, more slowly than the "touch signals" from a massage. Touch signals outrun pain. Therefore a massage, with signals traveling on A-beta nerves to the brain at 180-200 miles per hour, creates a sort of traffic jam at the spinal cord's pain gates.[4]

Pain management during massages

Massage therapy is sometimes uncomfortable: it can even be really painful to the one in pain; it may force you to practice pain reducing therapies, such as deep breathing or self hypnosis. However massage presents benefits, including increased mobility, that appear almost immediately. It is important to explain how you feel during treatment in order for the therapist to adjust pressure and movements, and find the best approach for you. Visualization and deep breathing, meditation music and perfumed oils are essential during massages in order to relax and mitigate any pain caused by pressure on injured areas. Essential oils and fragrant creams are pleasant and relaxing in addition to lubricating hand motion. Plain conversation with the therapist also helps as a distraction. You may be able to ask questions and learn something positive during the therapy; you will also discover that, if pain becomes too intense on one part of the body during the treatment, the human brain does not feel pain elsewhere. This is really important for people suffering from multiple injury sites. Pain may increase at one spot during massages but at the same time, you will probably not feel the pain elsewhere. It is important to select the right places for massages because pain is able to travel fast. As an example, neck muscles affect the shoulders, upper back and arms from shoulders to fingernails.

Massage techniques

Massage usually is based on three main strokes: effleurage (that is stroking) with the hand to relax and facilitate the blood and lymph flow; pressure with fingers on the nerves, and kneading with fingers and thumbs to relieve muscle tension and improve blood circulation. Other techniques include vibration, friction and percussion.

People in chronic pain may benefit from deep myofascial treatment, when the therapist wants to reach the fascia or tissue surrounding soft tissues, and from pressure for a few seconds on trigger points which are these nasty hard little muscular knots giving so much pain in areas away from the source of pain. Pressure on trigger points forces them to relax by depriving them of oxygen, but this pressure may require up to 40 pounds of weight which you calculate by pressing on your bathroom scale.[5] I find myofascial massage can be fairly painful at the time of the treatment, but it is highly beneficial to increase mobility.

Marg and Cynthia, my massage therapists

Margaret joined my team of caregivers when Christy, my regular massage therapist, went on maternity leave. Marg was trained as a chiropractor before becoming a massage therapist. She shares a clinic with my chiropractor and I used to hear her laughing with her clients when I visited my chiropractor. Of course she has worries like all of us, she lives alone with her dog and as I recently discovered, she gets pain in her arms from using her muscles to take care of her clients. This does not prevent her from finding joy in helping them to feel better. Her laugh is a sort of trademark. The first time she saw me, she asked me to show her my feet because she needed what she called "a road map". Touching feet allowed her to describe exactly my pain on the forehead, neck, shoulders and upper back. The road map was excellent and I did not have to describe my pain! Marg works on the pressure points found on the feet and on the rest of the body. She knows which parts of the body can be associated with the pressure points on the feet. She keeps surprising me and she has an extraordinary talent to understand the sources of the pain.

No need to tell her where it hurts since she finds it on her own! The treatment, especially the pressure on the foot, is painful even with mental training and deep breathing. A burning pain may also appear on the parts of the body which were massaged to get rid of trigger points and muscle spasms. However a few hours after the treatment the body feels wonderfully relaxed and becomes mobile again. It is important to enjoy this temporary well-being to the maximum because painless moments are a precious rarity no one wants to miss. I also receive massages from Cynthia who made of her clinic an oasis with candles and flowers. I feel much better each time I leave this extraordinary space.

Good results come from massaging the muscles forcing the body to eliminate the lactic acid crystals, from bonding and from being touched by strong and caring hands. These three components are a recipe for success.

Craniosacral therapy

This therapy is very gentle and recommended to decrease pain from headaches and TMJ. The therapist applies light pressure on the suture lines of the skull and on several other parts of the body. The goal is to balance the cerebrospinal fluid surrounding the brain and the spinal cord. This liquid goes from the head to the base of the spine; pain appears when the fluid is interrupted. I found this mysterious science very relaxing and I loved the light touch on the head even if my pain could increase even with gentle pressure. This therapy often decreases pain suffered by many people and should be tried even if results are not necessarily immediate and quickly recognizable. When I leave my therapist, after a craniosacral session, I feel lighter and more energetic. Craniosacral therapy has a remarkable positive impact on my mood.

Why not self-massages?

You should be able to massage up to a certain extent parts of your body on your own, except for the middle back, or you could ask a partner or a friend to do it or you could see a professional therapist. Massages provided by another person always give better results because they offer bonding and contact with caring and energetic hands. However it is a good idea to combine them with self-massages that give reasonably good results at no cost.

If you decide to try self-massage, try preparing the room with music and scent the air by heating essential oils. You will need also oil to pour on your hands and spread on the parts of the body to be massaged. I find sitting on the bed is the most comfortable place.

- You knead firmly from the base of one side of your neck to the top of your arm and back.

- You use all fingers and sweep them firmly 12 times from the center of the collarbones to the armpits to remove the body toxins. If you are a woman and if you have pain in the upper part of the body, you knead each breast a few times to detoxify the chest a bit more.

- You knead the arm from wrist to shoulder by using the opposite hand.

- Then with one or two hands you do an effleurage movement or you knead the legs from ankles to hips, one leg after the other; you go upward to encourage lymphatic drainage.

- You massage each hand with the other hand by pressing the thumb in a circular movement and you massage on the foot each sole by pressing with the thumb. In addition to this method,[6] you knead any parts of the body which are tense with spasms or trigger points, without causing any major additional pain which could be a sign you are too hard on the injured parts.

When you massage yourself, you may have also to use arms and shoulders which are tense and painful; pain will increase if you knead. You could manage this challenge by using one hand at a time and by pressing the other hand under the elbow of the arm which is kneading. If when kneading, even a light movement is too painful for the part getting the massage or for the arm that does the work, you should switch to effleurage. It is also more comfortable to massage the neck, the head and the face by lying down on the bed (eliminating the need to hold elbows up in the air without any support) or placing the elbows on a side table for support. These are the movements I prefer for the face: making gentle small circles; tapping lightly; using two fingers on each side of the face and firmly pulling the skin from the top of the nose to the cheeks and from the forehead to the sides towards the temples; with the thumb and the index, pinching the skin along the eyebrow and pulling the top skin slightly downwards toward the eye; pulling the bottom part of the ear down slightly. The movements on the forehead and the eyebrows are excellent to reduce headache pain on the forehead. For headaches on other parts of the head, including under the hair, I find pulling the skin to the sides, applying pressure or pulling the hair slightly very useful. Self-massage requires time and is more relaxing after a warm bath.

Lumps: lymph or cancer issues?

If you notice lumps on the breast, chest or armpits during your self-massaging session, they could be lymph nodes requiring better drainage and elimination of toxins; another possibility is cancer because women with chronic pain get cancer just like any other women. Chronic pain is exhausting and stressful for the body; this means bodies of women with chronic pain in theory are more at risk of getting cancer. Lumps **must** be reported immediately to a physician for further examination. Most lumps must be verified by a mammogram and an ultrasound; chances are they will be the result of muscle spasms pressing and preventing the lymphatic system from working properly. Still they should be checked to eliminate the possibility of breast cancer. Most physicians do not check breasts for cancer lumps more than once a year and they do not handle massages; so if there is a lump, you will probably be the one to feel it first and to worry about it for a few days until you get results from medical tests ordered by your physician. You may be told you should work harder on removing toxins from your body. The way to do this is by daily massaging the parts of the body where the lymph system is found, to activate elimination of toxins. When chronic pain seems to take over everything we do, regular check-ups by physicians, for issues other than pain, and an yearly mammography are not on the top sections of the priority list; however they should be maintained there with priorities. Yes, we have pain but this pain will not prevent cancer. So, please use common sense: Have any regular tests done and immediately report any anomalies.

Short history

Massage, from the Arabic word *massa*, means "to touch" and is mentioned in a Chinese text dated to 2598 B.C. Ancient temples in India show Buddha having massages. The Greeks as well as the Romans had massages as part of their common practices for well-being. Swedish massage, a form of deep massage of the joints and muscles, started in the early 1800s and spread in Europe and the United States.[7] The theory of Per Henrik Ling, the gymnast who developed Swedish massage, was that massage was a type of passive exercise to help heal.[8] Swedish massage is very popular now because it treats the entire body and I was told that it prevents medical disorders; Californian massage was born in Big Sur (California) in 1970 and brings comfort and relaxation with its fluid and ongoing movements.[9] Warm stones can be used with the Swedish and Californian massages to bring additional comfort and a connection with nature. Japanese forms of massage cover 5

000 years of history and include numerous ways to press or pull with the hands, the arms, the elbows and the knees.

Rolfing is a form of deep muscular massage developed in the 1930s by a biochemist called Ida Rolf. The goal is to restore the body to a natural position when emotions force the client to take unnatural postures hardening tissues and restricting natural movement. Rolfing brings good results to many people but, because it involves deep pressure, some find it too painful. Advice from your pain specialist is recommended if you are interested in rolfing because this treatment is a very deep massage.

Any one can benefit from massage: athletes, runners, healthy people active in all sorts of sports, tense people of any ages, the ill and of course those suffering from chronic pain, such as back pain or migraines. Massage is even excellent as a mental therapy: It provides an opportunity for clients to communicate pain to a compassionate therapist. Even if massages are painful, they offer a feeling of well-being which may last for two-three hours or one day or even one week. In my case the break from pain massage provides, is measured in hours, not in days. Massage also offers a precious opportunity to receive some human and caring touch.

ACUPRESSURE, A WIDELY USED THERAPY

Pressure with hands and elbows on specific points in the body is called acupressure. This therapy combines massage and acupuncture. This technique is close to acupuncture but the therapist uses fingers, palms and sometimes elbows, instead of needles, to knead, manipulate and massage acupressure points where blocked nerve energy causes soreness. These points, where organic disorders are said to be reflected, are slightly painful; they are also found on about one third of the 365 acupuncture points, mainly on bodily organs, along the spine and on the forehead.[10] In Chinese medicine energy (called *chi*) is said to flow along channels in the body. Disease follows when the flow of *chi* is blocked. Nerve energy or *chi* is released by pressure on points found on these channels. This pressure lasts from thirty seconds to twenty minutes.[11] You stop pressing when soreness begins to fade.

Japanese therapists practice shiatsu (*shi* for finger and *atsu* for pressure) and apply very deep pressure on a point progressively for a few seconds. They use their hands but also their elbows, knees and feet to work on a client, and they incorporate passive stretching and meditation into the therapy.[12] Shiatsu is said to restore normal flowing of *chi*, to rebalance the life forces and to relax the body and the mind. It may be painful because of the amount of finger pressure that is applied. However the goal is to relieve pain, ease off stiffness in the muscles and improve the nervous, circulatory and immune systems.[13] In plain language this means shiatsu reduces anxiety, stress, chronic pain, migraines, asthma and insomnia in addition to other common problems such as, for example, cramps.

Acupressure is not dangerous and can be learned by the one in pain even if some points, for instance on the back, are impossible to reach. A friend can also learn and help you in stimulating each point out. Acupressure may of course be too painful because it involves pressure on injuries and you will know if pain decreases after the treatment. If it is too painful or if it does not bring any benefits, it is time to try another therapy.

Acupressure works well for pain because it distracts

the nervous system and promotes well-being. The nerve impulses carrying the message for firm touch go faster than the ones carrying pain messages, and prevent them from going up the spinal cord. The therapeutic and relaxing effects of acupressure last after the time of treatment[14] even if the pressure must be repeated on a regular basis to reduce chronic pain.

REFLEXOLOGY, A TOOL FOR HEALING

Reflexology is based on the principle that small parts of the body can be used to treat the whole and on the idea that the body itself has the ability to heal by itself. When properly offered, reflexology treats chronic pain, breathing disorders and numerous other issues, such as heart and lung problems. The word "properly" is essential: many people receive a sort of foot massage and call it reflexology when the real treatment is something highly different. If you belong to this group of people in pain, it is not too late to look for a therapist with more experience. However, please remember that reflexology, in the same way as massage and acupressure, can be painful with different degrees because your resistance to pain and your therapist's training are unique. Of course you must not refuse reflexology because you have just read I found it painful: everybody is different in the experience of pain. Moreover practicing deep breathing techniques helps you to face the world when you hurt.

The ten zones

All important acupressure points are located on the hands and feet where all parts of the body can be mapped.

Reflexology therapists do firm massages on these points to bring changes in other parts of the body such as neck or head, to restore balance in the body and free up energy pathways. The body is divided into ten vertical zones including five on the right side and five on the left. Parts on the foot and the hand found in one zone affect other parts of the body in that same zone. Nerve endings for a specific zone on the foot and the hand, if treated by pressure, will relax and bring relief to other parts of the body within the same zone since the entire body is represented in the feet and since reflexology stimulates healing in the whole body.

Crushing the beads

Reflexologists believe that abnormal crystal deposits of material form at nerve endings in the feet and interfere with circulation. They say that the pressure they apply crushes these crystals into a form that may be removed by the blood; circulation improves and the body then becomes relaxed.[15] This treatment has nothing to do with foot massages or with rubbing feet. Pressure on these crystal beads can be awfully painful and some people do not have a pain threshold high enough to go through this treatment. Fortunately mental exercises of visualization added to meditation music and total trust in your therapist's healing hands will allow you to receive a treatment which really helps to restore mobility; once momentary increased pain is managed. In addition, even if a better physical range can't be reached, you can concentrate on the thought that increasing pain will disappear as soon as the treatment is over. Even if the level of pain and range were the same after and before reflexology, just because pain increased during the session, you will feel better physically at the end of the treatment when pain goes back to the usual level after an increased peak. Since pain is a perception, we can learn how to take advantage of it, instead of fighting it, if there is some sort of comfort to get from it.

History

We can say reflexology is as old as our world: At Saqqarah, in Egypt, a 2330 B.C. fresco, found in Ankmahor's tomb, shows a physician practicing reflexology on another man; this therapy was also common in China many years ago. An American doctor, William Fitzgerald (1872-1942), developed the zone therapy and divided the body into 10 vertical zones; and a therapist, Eunice Ingham, who passed away in 1974 at the age of 85 year-old, is considered to be the founder of modern reflexology because, through her publications and hard work, she made this therapy accepted by the medical profession.[16] Reflexology is usually practiced on feet but can be done also on hands where the thumb is connected to the head and skull, and the bottom of the thumb, to the neck, with the side of the hand, below the thumb, to the side to the spine.[17] You too can apply reflexology on your hands after being shown how to do it.

CHIROPRACTIC CARE,
ALWAYS THE KING OF UNIVERSAL DEBATE

This therapy is the universal monarch of all debates on care to the spinal cord. Chiropractic is the second most widely recognized medical profession in the world, with traditional western medicine being the first.[18] In addition it offers excellent relief for back pain, even if the adjustment or correction to the position of spinal vertebrae must sometimes be done on a regular basis. Chiropractic is commonly criticized by conventional medicine especially in cases involving the neck.

The word chiropractic comes from a Greek word meaning "done by hand" and the one who invented chiropractic was a Canadian grocer born in Ontario called Daniel Palmer who moved to the States. In 1895 he manipulated the neck of a deaf person who managed to recover hearing. A new medical profession was born. Chiropractic care is given now by specialized and knowledgeable therapists using mainly their hands to give relief from pain and discomfort by pushing, pulling and turning. This treatment can be combined with other methods of health care.

Chiropractic adjustments or manipulations help correct malfunctioning areas of the spine and other joints to decrease pain and increase mobility. The therapy involves using mainly hands to move a joint a little past its current range of motion; this causes the vertebrae to pop back into place and the manipulation can produce a popping sound when gases escaping from two joints is released.[19] These treatments allow better range; they also free the nerves from disruptions caused by displaced or misaligned vertebrae; in addition they reset neurological patterns affecting muscle tone and the way pain signals are processed in the spinal cord.[20] I believe contacts from caring hands and conversations, where people in pain discuss physical challenges with compassionate therapists, are very therapeutic. Chiropractors may also apply heat or ice, use massage, ultrasound or gentle electrotherapy. My personal experience is that manipulation is not painful if we are relaxed and trust the therapist. Chiropractic treats numerous health issues, such as headaches, colds, asthma, heart, respiratory and intestinal problems if these disorders result from abnormal nerve functions; most adjustments are done on the spine which is the center of the nervous system. You understand that in these treatments having an impact on the nerves, the relationship between client and chiropractor must be excellent to allow the client to relax during the treatment and to make the manipulation possible.

Dr. Darrell, my Chiropractor

In this area also I visited a few chiropractors before meeting Darrell (his clients use his first name) who was able to show me the benefits offered by chiropractic to people experiencing chronic pain. Muscle spasms caused by physical injuries pull joints out of place; when the joints are not in the right place, they create even more muscle spasms... and the one in pain gets pain from this vicious circle from the muscle spasms, from the nerves not working properly and from the joints being out of place. When this scenario takes place in the neck or the spine, it can affect any part of the body, since the nerves controlling the body go through the neck. If the nerves and muscles in the neck do not work properly, the shoulders are out of balance, with one higher than the other, the arms seem to lose energy and be made of marshmallow, the back and the body in general may burn for no apparent reason, one hip can become lower than the other one, with an immediate consequence of making one leg shorter than the other, and the head may house constant headaches.

So, several years ago, I wondered why it was so easy for me to trip for absolutely no reason; at the same time I decided to put my hair up in a bun. This desire for a new hairstyle was a great lesson: it taught me it was about impossible to use my hands above the head and it showed me on the mirror my shoulders would not stay even. I decided to leave my hair floating on the shoulders since it would hide so beautifully my shoulder line and I ended up in Dr. Darrell's clinic with a recommendation from my physician who was unable to help me with my Christmas tree look caused by uneven shoulders. I still end up in Darrell's clinic each week but the symptoms decrease for a few hours after each treatment and this is an improvement. Bonding with someone I trust and getting chiropractic care each week from this person help me a lot mentally and also physically; the feeling of improved well-being that I get when I leave the clinic, is a great moral boost even if I know the physical improvement will disappear during the day or the night. I load my brain with these feelings of doing better and when it hurts again, I pull them out from my mental bank account and tell myself soon I will visit again Dr. Darrell's clinic.

Requirements for a successful therapy

Many people, including the healthy, can benefit from physical therapy. Unfortunately we tend to judge any medical treatment in the 30 seconds following the beginning of the conversation with the therapist, so we tell our body it is not going to work if the therapist does not seem to have any affinities with us or does not succeed to make us feel comfortable. Sometimes we even believe the visit will be a massive waste of time if we do not like the receptionist. Of course this brings no positive results. It is probably the same for many therapists who judge their clients as soon as they step in the room, instead of assessing the injuries.... because many people still think the pain could be "only" in the head. Here is a quick tip to recognize this type of situation: if you find yourself explaining pain is real instead of, for example, showing how pain affects your life. Again, if there is no affinity between the client and the therapist, the treatment will not work. Good connections between the client and the medical professional are always important but here, with chiropractic, they are essential because of the risks commonly perceived as high in situations involving the nervous system. If the client believes the treatment could damage the body even more, the therapy is not going to work even if the treatment is excellent because of the mind's impact on the natural painkilling agents found in the nervous system. So closeness and trust are very important for chiropractic to heal the body.

Unfair perception

In the 1950s and 1960s the American Medical Association launched a public relations campaign against chiropractors. In 1986 in Wilke v. AMA, the American Medical Association was convicted in federal court of being "the largest professional violator of the Sherman antitrust laws" after a three-decade long campaign to discredit and undermine the field of chiropractic. A permanent injunction order against the American Medical Association by Federal Court Judge Susan Getzendammer was published in January 1988 in the *Journal of the American Medical Association* and other rulings on the case appeared in following issues. The three chiropractors who brought the suit against a defense supported by a $ 6 million U. S. legal budget, requested no damages because they did not want financial gain to be perceived as the reason for the litigation. The chiropractors only asked for the ruling to be published in the defendant's own journal.[21] Fortunately the hostility between chiropractors and medical doctors is decreased today.[22]

However, physicians warning clients about risks of paralysis or internal bleeding during chiropractic treatment is still very common. No one seems to remember these unfortunate outcomes would occur only in the context of specific preexisting medical conditions. Our medical culture still encourages the use of conventional medicine over alternative medicine, including chiropractic, despite the fact that the latter returns individual control to clients and is effective in cures when traditional western medicine fails.

ELECTRICAL STIMULATION, ONE OF THE MOST ANCIENT THERAPIES

That electricity has healing properties is not a new discovery. Ancient Greeks used electric eels to relieve the pain of headaches and gout, and their physicians discussed the most appropriate fish to be used. In the 19th century hand-generated electricity was used to relieve pain and about one century later in 1965 the gate control theory was developed by Melzac. It was then demonstrated that electricity played a part in reducing pain. It was realized that electrical stimulation seemed to close the pain gate and jam the pain messages in the spinal cord while confusing the brain so that it cannot recognize pain signals any more. This is the reason why transcutaneous electrical nerve stimulation (TENS) breaks a muscle spasm by creating another spasm and can bring some relief.[23]

Benefits

Electrotherapy can be useful to reducing muscle and nerve pain, increasing blood circulation and, as many people believe, elevating levels of endorphins, our body's natural painkillers. Other wonderful news to share with you: TENS is not painful! It produces only a tingling sensation. In technical terms, it is low-intensity (it doesn't hurt) and high-frequency (stimulation is about 100 times per second).[24] Chiropractors sometimes use this stimulation.

How it works

The small battery-operated TENS machine is about the size of a small adult hand. It sends a painless electric current through the skin and into the soft tissues. Electrodes are placed on the skin, usually above the pain. The wire between these electrodes and the battery-powered unit can be hidden in the clothes and the unit can be hooked to any piece of clothing around the waist. Users manage intensity, speed and depth of simulation themselves and the machine can be rented. If it effectively decreases your pain, you may wish to buy one. The idea of renting one first will show you if you belong to the 30 to 40 percent of people who get relief from it. The machine costs a few hundred dollars and you should not spend so much money if it does not help you. You continue your normal day of work even if you carry this small device because it is very easy to hide it in your clothes.

The more time spent with the machine, the better the results. Normal activities can be maintained while using the machine, except of course activities that would damage any electrical appliance, like a shower. Of course your therapist should make a recommendation before you use the machine because some people, such as those who have a pacemaker, should not use it.

I tried using the TENS a few times. The last time I had a muscle knot on a shoulder, that, for several days, had prevented me from moving my head freely. I borrowed the unit from my chiropractor, two days or so before Christmas, but realized after a few days I would not get much help from it. The tingling sensation kept reminding me I had massive injury of the neck, shoulder and back; even if it did not cause any major additional pain, the tingling was not pleasant; in addition, the affected area was too large for the machine to be helpful. I had to move the electrodes because the pain was not localized. The exercise turned into a race between the electrodes and the trigger points that would always appear outside the stimulated area. I decided my body did not need this race. Of course people with widely spread pain may benefit from a dorsal column stimulator surgically implanted in the epidural space near the spinal cord or even in the brain.[25] I decided not to risk surgery.

OSTEOPATHY, A HIDDEN SCIENCE

Osteopathy is a treatment method based on bone manipulation, in contrast to chiropractic, where manipulation almost exclusively is performed on the vertebrae. Osteopathic adjustments may be made on almost any bone in the body. Osteopathy was developed by Dr. Andrew Taylor Still in the late 1800s in the United States. Dr. Still believed that by manipulating the bones, he could stimulate the nervous system and the blood circulation.[26] Early osteopathy was based solely on cracking joints but this practice was highly criticized by the medical profession. The school of osteopathy Dr. Still founded was open to blacks and women, an admission policy that was very unusual in the United States at the time. Dr. Still died in 1917, subsequently his followers came to include medications and other conventional therapies in their treatments, thus gaining the acceptance of conventional physicians. Today osteopaths are fully licensed physicians allowed to prescribe medications. There is no difference today between osteopathy and conventional medicine, except that osteopaths tend to have a more holistic approach and to treat the entire person rather than diseases.

PHYSIOTHERAPY, AN ESSENTIAL THERAPY

Physiotherapy is a part of health care which emphasizes the use of physical approaches in the prevention, treatment and rehabilitation of a disability. Physiotherapists are trained to prevent, identify and alleviate movement dysfunction. Physiotherapy decreases pain and improves the range of movement and strength.[27] Any one in pain and willing to improve should consult a physiotherapist because pain affects movement and movement affects pain. The therapist works on soft tissues by teaching specific exercises designed to prevent and/or heal physical disorders, by using electrical stimulation and by massaging muscles. The client will receive advice on exercises to do at home. The therapy will be of benefit only to those who are committed enough to play an active role in their rehabilitation and well-being.

Physiotherapists can also use hot and cold pads to treat muscles and trigger points. These pads are not expensive and they are very easy to enjoy at home. They can be painful for the first minutes but relief usually comes quickly. They can be used alternately or you may select a single type if you prefer. Warm pads stimulate release of endorphins, increase blood circulation, are comforting after an exercise, before or after a therapy such as massage, or any other time; they increase range of motion and quickly reduce muscle tension. Cold pads also stimulate endorphin release. In addition, they reduce muscle spasms, pain and inflammation. In one study cold therapy reduced migraine pain in 80 percent of people in pain.[28] These magic bags, made of beans or smaller seeds, can be cooled in the deep freezer or warmed in the microwave oven. They work almost immediately. My bag travels with me and goes each day to the office. We never know when magic bags will be helpful and we must be ready to use them if needed. Towels coming from the dryer or the deep freezer offer the same benefits as the pads. Ice packs or hot-water bottles or electric blankets can also be used. Cold is good when the skin feels hot for any reason such as from inflammation of the nerves or from arthritis. You should make sure you do not use intense heat which can increase sunburn pain caused by inflammation of the nervous system. Saunas and hot baths are other means of gaining the benefits coming from heat.

Why do warm and cold pads decrease pain so quickly? They work so well because sensory nerves are highly responsive to temperature. Cold pads prevent the nerve from carrying information very well. The nerve temporarily loses its ability to bring pain signals to the brain. Heat and cold, both close the spinal cord's pain gate.[29] You select cold or warm temperature according to your personal preferences, or any credible characteristic of the particular injury or disease.

KINESIOTHERAPY, ANOTHER
CONCEALED THERAPY

This is a complex word for a very important and essential component of your pain management activities. "Kinetic" means: Of or relating to the motion of material bodies and the forces and energy associated therewith.[30] "Therapy" is the treatment of any physical disorder by medical or physical means, so all in all, to make it simple, kinesiotherapy is: improvement through movement. Any one suffering from chronic pain knows how painful it is to get up in the morning after a period of time without any movement. Pain seems to multiply after a rest and the simplest movement can become a huge challenge bringing tears to the eyes.

A kinesiotherapist is a health care professional who, under the direction of a physician, treats the effects of disease and injuries, through the use of therapeutic exercise and education.[31] All in all, you want to include this specialist of the human movement in your circle of therapists. Kinesiology began in 1943 after World War II when injured soldiers had to receive corrective physical reconditioning before going back to active fighting after their injuries. The corrective therapy based on therapeutic exercises in rehabilitation was renamed kinesiotherapy in 1987.

Kinesiotherapy helps the ones with chronic pain to maximize their strength, coordination, range of motion and mobility. It can also be preventive in that it teaches one to eliminate any movements that hurt the body. It may also include massages and advice for a better lifestyle and for prevention of possible painful conditions. Kinesiotherapy is commonly used to treat back pain by rehabilitation and education on good posture. Sometimes unconscious habits damage the body and must be changed to improve general well-being. Quite often pain and stress force me to move with tight muscles and to look like a diving board; relaxed movements can be learned to reduce pain and this is an ongoing challenge. Other times the environment forces us to develop a bad posture. Do you have to lift up the eyes or bend down the neck to read the computer screen? If yes, you should make sure the top of your screen is just in front of your eyes. Bending the neck or looking up is surprisingly hard job for the neck supporting the head. We may need assistance from a kinesiotherapist to make sure our environment is as friendly as possible for our body.

EXERCISES, A THERAPY
FILLED WITH LOVE AND HATE

Most of us hate the word "exercise!" So, please join the club! Physical exercises take time and they are scary because they may increase the pain before bringing improvement. A strong mind to persevere and the will to feel better are the starting point for something physical. Some exercises are very easy, for example stretching or following, with your eyes, your finger moving from right to left in front of your nose. We do not know how moving the eyes can lead to a decrease in pain but it is believed this exercise imitates what happens during the rapid eye-movement sleep, and helps the body to digest traumas and bad memories.[32] Try it! It forces you to relax by focusing on your finger.

Benefits

Exercises are essential to recovery because they make us stronger. They improve the overall function of the brain made of flesh and blood; they improve blood circulation and, please don't forget, according to my therapists the brain uses 20 percent of all oxygen pumped by the heart, therefore any improvement in circulation enhances brain function by giving the brain extra oxygen, nutrients and glucose fuel. Exercises increase output of an important brain hormone called "nerve growth factor," that helps brain cells to function at peak efficiency; they also improve the metabolism of the brain by encouraging nutrients to enter the brain and by speeding the removal of toxins. Because the brain controls the pain, exercising the body, with such a positive effect on the fitness of the brain, is very important.[33]

In addition, exercise stimulates the mechanism of pleasure in the brain,[34] develop serotonin and endorphins (the body natural painkillers), release tension built up in the muscles, prevent trigger points, strengthen muscles and bones. A good supply of serotonin is essential because it has even a greater effect on the mind than the endorphins, where impact is mainly physical; in addition, the serotonin boost from exercise persists long after the session is done.[35] If you exercise, you also increase your levels of norepinephrine, the adrenal neurotransmitter boosting mood and energy. The amount of norepinephrine created by exercise helps to activate a counterattack against pain.[36]

Exercise also helps stabilize estrogen levels (the sex hormone interfering with serotonin). Unstable levels of this hormone may partly explain the fact that chronic pain is more common in women than in men.[37]

Exercise helps to restore muscle flexibility and to reduce pain by giving additional nourishment to muscles and by increasing blood blow in injured areas. Finally, exercise helps one to lose weight. This can be crucial for people suffering from pain in the supporting parts of the body, such as the spine. Would you agree that exercises seem to become increasingly attractive as you get informed on their benefits?

Exercise should be part of a daily routine. A good exercise session can be as little as 20-30 minutes, if the workout is intense enough to raise the heartbeat by 50 percent and if you complete with other activities allowing you to move inside and outside the home.[38] Don't forget your brain needs the help provided by brisk exercise! Even 20 minutes of exercise 3 times per week can reduce pain. One of the most important points is to exercise to the limits of our abilities on a regular basis.[39] In my experience, going beyond these limits can increase pain and when I feel my neck starting to burn, I know I have reached my limit.

Exercises combined with pleasure

You should combine several types of exercise in your program, making an interesting and pleasant regimen. I find it crucial to structure exercising so it is interesting. This is possible if we exercise with other people,[40] if we breathe properly, or do a form of meditation, or listen to music or watch a movie during exercises. The nature of exercises will depend on the type and location of pain. You should get an exercise program from your doctor or from a therapist because you do not want to conduct ill-advised experiments with your body. However only you know how much to push your body, how long and how hard you should exercise. Sometimes it takes a few hours for pain to set in after an exercise session and for you to understand that you overdid it. Exercising is good; increasing pain for a long time is bad; becoming even stiffer and getting a burning pain are very bad. If you develop persistent discomfort after exercising, you should adjust your program. You will know what to do. Common sense is essential.

Exercise also is conducive to having a good rest at night. Sleeping is not at all a waste of time! I mention it because I thought it was a total waste until I had the car accident and realized a good night of sleep would help me to keep pain under control. Sleep helps to regenerate physical energy, to reorganize our learning and to manage emotions.[41] Before the accident, I would spend evenings and numerous first hours of the day in my office at home, reading, sorting out parts of articles on my computer, putting together ideas, writing, proofreading... and I would see these activities as real benefits taken from limiting sleep. I still do all these activities but I have learned to slow down (I am still learning!) and to see sleep as a partner in my pain management plan. Pain told me about the importance of many things and now I have on my priorities list: walks outside along the river before bed time, smelling rose bushes in the garden during the summer, and sleeping at night.

Exercise does not have to be painful, even if the opposite (the "work through the pain" or the "keep going in spite of pain") is claimed by several private sport clinics making revenues from the ones with chronic pain, especially when this income comes from direct payment from car insurances. So, do not deal harshly with your body when it is already suffering from pain! In addition, what would you gain from suffering more? Simply nothing except for increased number of thoughts about suicide or other subjects of a depressing nature!

Some exercises are very relaxing and give one a feeling of well-being. These are the ones you need because if you feel good, you will exercise on a regular basis. Among these ones, I would put walking in warm pools and walking briskly in nature. Warm pools are often found in hospitals, clinics and rehabilitation centers. Doing any exercise in warm water relaxes the muscles and gives a better range of movement. You should check in your area to see whether you can access a warm pool.

Walking while surrounded by nature is a good exercise especially if you go at a brisk pace because the kind of exercise stimulating endorphin release is aerobic.[42] Nature offers numerous distractions with countless plants, flowers, and small wild animals. It is possible to forget the pain and increase the pace if our mind is busy enjoying nature. Your heart rate will increase without you noticing it. Another activity to recommend is swimming because this exercise allows all the muscles to work without putting stress on the joints. Dancing is of course one of my favorite physical activities. I have joined the Orchesis Dance Group at the University of Alberta (Edmonton). Dance allows me to connect with others and create something beautiful. This helps me to forget my pain.

Yoga and tai chi are other excellent physical activities which are discussed in the chapter on psychology since they are closely connected to mental therapies. Sports can be fun even for people with chronic pain! One rule: You stop if pain increases or if your body sends you signals, such as dizziness, to tell you are overdoing it.

Simple activities

Some exercises involve only changes to positions, such as sitting after standing or standing after sitting because changing positions frequently prevents muscles from freezing and tensing. It is of course impossible to list all the exercises that could be considered for specific medical issues. However here are a few common ones.

One exercise suggested to ease headaches is the head roll, which stretches tense muscles. You sit and bring down the chin to the chest, then you slowly circle your head to the left, drop it back, bring it to the right and back to the chest.

Exercises that I find useful for relaxing the neck and easy enough to do after waking up, are to stay in bed on the back, a roll under the neck, and to turn the head to right and to left; to sit on a chair, to turn the head all the way to the right, to return the head to normal and to turn the head all the way to the left. As you will see, head has more range when the body rests on a bed because in this position, the neck does not have to support the head.

Another common exercise for the neck is to sit on a chair, to tilt the head to the right towards the shoulder (in other words, try to touch the shoulder with the ear); to go back to normal with straight head; to tilt head to the left towards the shoulder. A good tension reliever for the neck is to sit on a chair, clasp both hands on top of the neck to the back and push the head against the hands.

Physicians do not agree with the use of cervical collars that hold the neck rigidly in one position and provide support. One of the negative impacts comes from the neck muscles, already tense, tightening up even more because of the lack of movement. Specialists now tend to oppose the use of these collars; they claim collars make muscles weaker and stiffer when they are already stiff by themselves to protect the neck bones in cases of injury. However hard collars are essential to hold unstable vertebrae in the neck and to prevent any complications.

Several exercises for the jaws can improve elasticity of the muscles and reduce TMJ symptoms. Some easy exercises are to open the mouth wide and close it slowly; or to move the bottom jaw from side to side, back and forth; to curl up the tongue, to place it on the roof of the mouth to open and close the mouth with the tongue in this position. These exercises, repeated several times a day for as long as possible, have helped me to decrease this embarrassing clicking noise caused by opening the jaws. At its most, it was just like hearing someone slamming a door. Now the noise has disappeared, and I feel a lot more comfortable if I eat in public. However my TMJ condition makes any jaw exercises extremely painful and I suggest to verify with a professional which exercises would be the best for your condition.

Other exercises are becoming popular and can be also considered. Pilates was once used mainly by dancers who wanted to get stronger but it is now taught in major cities to any one interested in conditioning exercises. Videos are also available for those who prefer to learn at home. Pilates is an example of a variety of conditioning techniques that strengthen muscles and have a meditative effect; it is especially useful in cases of chronic pain because it does not stretch the joints, and it offers stress relief.[43]

Simplify ergonomics

Other exercises involve simplified or modified physical activities in every day life.

Preventive measures should also be followed to fight bad habits. For example, it is recommended that one bends the knees while lifting objects. If you are used to standing for a long time, you may put one foot up on a bar or a box and alternate feet; or try to sit for a change. When you sit at a desk, use a straight and hard chair supporting your back; sit with your knees horizontal to your hips (this may involve putting feet on a support); put a round pillow or rolled up towel between the chair and your middle back; get up by putting one foot in front of the other and shifting your weight forward. When you work at a computer screen, adjust it to make sure you do not have to look down or up at the screen; imagine a horizontal line between your screen and your eyes and make the necessary adjustments on your screen to obtain this line. Books under the screen are great to raise the height of the screen. If you sit for a long time, think of shifting your weight by crossing your legs or moving your weight to one hip or the other, or even get up for short walks.

Another common bad habit is to bend over while doing something; so, please stand up. Another one is to stretch to reach something high and out of reach. In this case, you should use a stool or small ladder and (in order to add support to your back by tightening abdominal muscles) breathe out when you lift. Also please carry heavy objects close to the front of your body. When driving put the seat close to the pedals and make sure your knees are level with your hips. Although this can indeed increase the possibility of being hit more strongly by your air bag, it can relax your leg muscles and improve your vision without straining your neck and arms.[44]

Living with chronic pain forces you to reassess your habits and to find solutions that increase comfort. Sometimes very simple activities are useful but we cannot expect miracles. Daily exercises have not helped me to bend my back; however I learned positions allowing me to function better. I solve the issue of cleaning the bathtub by using liquid body soap and by removing the last trace of the bath when I am still in the tub; everything shines when I leave the tub. Hugging and kissing can be challenging. I learned to hug my young children when they stood up on the stairs while I sat in front of them. I had to make sure they did not push my head back even when we played. A great way to hug with no danger to the neck is to roll and hug them on the floor.

My mind is still kept busy solving all sorts of physical problems caused by the body. At the end when the mind and the body teach me how to handle certain positions, I feel stronger. The mind finds creative solutions and is always there to support the body made stronger by exercise.

LIGHT THERAPY, A SURPRISING TREATMENT

Have you noticed how a brisk walk in the outdoors reduces pain? Or how it feels good to take sunlight in winter? Or how shorter days increase depression? These situations share something they have in common: the impact of natural light on the body and the mind.

Many believe that one of the most important issues in treating chronic pain is the levels of the neurotransmitter serotonin. Low levels are thought to be inadequate to create useful levels of serotonin, making us more vulnerable to pain and influencing the onset of migraines, depression and fibromyalgia. Light therapy is used to ensure a good supply of serotonin. Light is thought to be needed for the body to switch from melatonin production at night to serotonin production during the day. Melatonin initiates and maintains sleep but, if its production continues during the day due to lack of light, it decreases the availability of serotonin. Apparently this opens the door to lethargy, depression, need for sugar, reduced libido.... and this lowers the pain threshold as well as increases the felt presence of all existing pain.[45] So, to stay indoors is not the best.

Even in winter when it is cold, it is a good idea to wear warm clothes and take the sun during a walk. This is especially important for women who already experienced significantly reduced levels of serotonin from the middle to the end of their menstrual cycle.

What about artificial light? Full-spectrum light, called grow light because it stimulates growth of plants, must be at least 2,500 lux to trigger release of serotonin. Standard indoors light must be at least 10,000 lux to give the same benefits.[46] Unfortunately this amount of light can strain unprotected eyes and is not recommended unless managed by a therapist with experience in this area. Much research needs to take place in the field of light therapy because we do not fully understand how natural and full-spectrum lights stimulate increased longevity and trigger certain biochemical reactions, including the release of serotonin.

DIET, A LONG TERM COMPANION

This book does not have to be read from the beginning to the end and you may decide to start anywhere. If you believe nutrition involving body chemistry is a difficult field, please do not panic and come back to this section when you need it.

We are what we eat. This means food has an impact on our physical and mental health as well as on our behaviour. In other words, if you eat much fast food, your brain and your body do not receive the quality of nutrition obtained by diets relying more on freshly prepared foods. However the goal here is not to force you to analyze everything you eat. Hippocrates, the ancient Greek physician who lived in 400 B.C., is well known for having said foods are remedies and remedies are foods.[47] Therefore eating should be mindful and reflective thought should be used if you want eating to help you to be at peace with pain.

Certain foods are thought to decrease pain and inflammation, calm nerves and influence brain chemistry. Of course, food is also known to give us energy, which is a source of life. The ideal is to maximize intake of useful energy while making sure as little as possible of our own energy is spent on damaging our body. Certain types of food, such as alcohol, may damage the stomach, decrease energy and lower the amount of oxygen going to the brain, therefore causing inflammation on internal organs and preventing both intake and uptake of several nutrients.[48] This means we should be selective about the foods we want to eat if we wish to prevent illness and additional pain. When energy is spent on activities, it should be replaced in order for us to have adequate reserves for our needs.

Not overeating or increasing your weight is important because extra weight often brings additional pain. Euphoria can be obtained from comfort food such as chocolate and pastries, but this "high" increases muscle tension and carrying stored fat makes your muscles work harder.[49] Eating slowly, relaxing and sitting in a quiet place during a meal facilitate digestion. Medications may bring changes to your diet, for example some of them may push you to develop a taste for sugar. The antidepressants seem especially prone to this.

It is good to know a medication's secondary effects if this medication is to be taken for a long time. There will be then no surprise for the user who will be able to make a better decision on taking or not taking the medication, and on adjusting daily diet according to the secondary effects. Some medications such as antidepressants and anti-inflammatories may force you to drink a lot of water because one main side effect from these types of medications is dry mouth. Opioids may cause constipation that you can reduce by eating fibers, cashew nuts and licorice. Drinking water between meals is also essential because deshydratation increases levels of stress.[50] Injuries having a major impact on muscles may also significantly modify your dietary needs. Chronic pain can demand dietary changes, for example, if you suffer from a TMJ issue, steak, raw vegetables and any hard or chewy food may increase pain. Several head injuries will make soft food more attractive. The diet to follow should be studied to make sure it does not bring any additional stress or pain to the body.

Diet is often perceived as a selection of foods to lose weight, something almost as awful as the pain. We prefer to see diet as a strategy to increase energy and decrease pain. In Asia nutrition is viewed as a natural way to prevent disease. Our meaning of diet is similar to the Asian understanding.

Diet is important because deficiencies in the muscles make them more susceptible to spasm, and diet can reduce these deficiencies. In addition, a good diet increases the stress tolerance of the muscles. Stress is an important determinant of the experience of chronic pain, and diets that reduce stress are recommended. Salt, white sugar, artificial flavorings and colors, preservatives and alcohol should all be avoided.

The foregoing restrictions notwithstanding, numerous pleasant diets are possible to accommodate various tastes and needs. The food you decided to eat will depend on your personal taste and will be appropriate as long as it includes the six necessary classes of nutrients: vitamins, minerals, enzymes, fats, proteins and carbohydrates. An interesting approach to nutrition is to divide foods into *yin* products including drinks, fruits, cheese, milk, sweet, sour and hot foods, and into *yang* products including animal products and cereals. According to this approach, good nutrition is a matter of balancing *yin* and *yang* foods. Too much of one type (*yin* or *yang*) or too much of both is said to lead to chronic pain by increasing possibilities of developing cancer, arteriosclerosis, muscular issues and nervousness.[51] The vegetarian diet is becoming increasingly popular because it is a useful preventative of medical problems with the heart and arteries. In addition, carbohydrates -pasta, rice, bread- have a calming effect on nerves.

Another approach to nutrition holds that one does well to choose foods that boost the health of the brain, thereby controlling the pain. According to this view, a good diet for the brain eliminates fat. The logic behind this holds that the brain is composed of fat; if a dietary fat (loaded with harmful free radical molecules that speed up oxidation) is followed on a regular basis, the brain tissues can simply die from oxidation. When brain cells are lost, our ability to manage pain is reduced. Dietary fat also damages blood circulation in the brain. In addition, the anti-pain diet should be loaded with nutrients from whole grains, vegetables, fruits, soy products, nonfat dairy products and beans.[52] A vegetarian diet is excellent because it does not include animal fats; the Mediterranean diet with olive oil and antioxydants from fruits and vegetables is also excellent. Antioxydants protect against free radicals damaging the body.

NUTRITIONAL THERAPY, ANOTHER PRIORITY

Some nutrients, more than others, have a profound impact on pain, and the combination of ancient and modern nutritional remedies seem to work very well. For example, serotonin blocks the perception of pain in the brain and reduces release of the pain-carrying Substance P secreted in the spinal column in response to pain signals from nerves. Serotonin also helps to improve mood, to regulate the sleep cycle, and to increase blood vessel elasticity. Pain is more tolerable when we are not depressed and sleep better. When blood vessels are flexible, they do not leak blood so much and they cause less painful irritation.

Serotonin is made in the body from an amino acid called tryptophan, common in many foods we eat. People in pain need tryptophan. A very popular medication increasing serotonin levels is called Prozac. Elavil ©/ Amitriptyline, an anti-depressant facilitating sleep, is also a medication increasing the bioavailability of serotonin. Foods rich in tryptophan include turkey, chicken, cheddar cheese and other types of cheese, halibut, eggs, peanut and peanut butter, milk and soybeans, potatoes, rice, pasta, bread; the foods from this list that are rich in fat should of course be eaten in small quantities. These foods naturally stimulate the passage of tryptophan into the brain where it metabolizes to serotonin automatically. Tryptophan can be also taken as a medication or supplement. If you decide to acquire it from your diet, you should eat carbohydrates and sugar before you eat protein, otherwise your digestion will block the absorption of tryptophan.[53]

Strategies

The following strategies give good results:

- Eat nutrients that relieve inflammation causing pain.

- Eat nutrients that build pain-blocking serotonin helping to close the pain gates. This is important because pain forces the body to use its supply of serotonin and if the supply is not renewed, pain gets worse.

- Eat nutrients that boost the health of the brain and the nerves, because nerves help you to maintain a high pain threshold. When nerves are tired, pain hurts more even if the physical disorder is the same. So, to be at peace with pain, you must nurture the nerves as good old friends.

- Avoid dietary mistakes, such overeating or undereating. Such errors increase pain.[54]

Inflammation

Inflammation is a very complex process. The body floods the injured areas with blood providing extra white blood cells killing infection and bringing needed nutrients for healing. However part of this additional blood leaks out and causes swelling, pressure on pain nerves, stiffness and warmth. The leaking blood also releases chemicals sensitizing the area. Inflammation helps to heal, but it also causes pain and additional problems if the inflammation is constant. One of the chemicals rushed to the injured area is serotonin and this deprives the brain and spinal cord of the serotonin needed to close the pain gates. Pain increases with the shortage of serotonin in the brain and spinal cord. When pain increases, even more serotonin goes to the injured area. At the site of the inflammation, serotonin does not block the pain; it activates other chemicals, including the most important called prostaglandins which can help healing. Prostaglandins are made of nutrients coming from certain specific foods.[55]

Understanding the causes of pain, I now visualize prostaglandins healing the injured areas while I do deep breathing; this reduces pain. At peace with serotonin and prostaglandins, seeing them as little helpers, pain also seems to decrease. I took seven years to understand the activities surrounding my pain; I hope these lines will assist you in having a better knowledge of the processus your body is undergoing. Knowledge allows you to be in better control of your body and more at peace with pain.

Right fats decreasing pain and inflammation

Diets with the right fats, can also help to produce the good prostaglandins causing the blood to exit inflamed area quickly rather than building up in swollen tissues. The right kinds of fats for reducing inflammation include: EPA (eicosapentaenoic acid) from fish or supplements, GLA (gamma-linolenic acid) and ALA (alpha-linolenic acid, both from green vegetables and algae). Animal fat and some common vegetable cooking oils (including corn, sunflower and canola oils) are types of fat to avoid. You could substitute them with olive oil. Nonfat dairy products are acceptable. Meat and common vegetable oils should be eliminated because they contain enzymes that create a substance called arachidonic acid that encourages inflammation. Eating less fat will also fight pain by improving blood circulation that heals injuries and boosts the function of the brain. Did you know the brain uses 20 percent of all blood pumped by the heart?

Doses

Perfect doses of what would be the ideal amounts of nutrients and vitamins are highly controversial with some specialists saying overdoses can be dangerous. Once thought to be quite safe, questions have arisen over the advisability of high doses of water soluble vitamins. Large doses of vitamin C can cause kidney stones and massive doses of some B vitamins may cause nerve damage.

It is now suggested not to take more than the USRDA (U.S. Recommended Daily Allowance). It has long been known that vitamins A, D, E and K are fat soluble and can accumulate in the body. Overdoses of vitamin A can cause severe bone pain, headaches and nausea; a buildup of vitamin E can give headaches.[56] Your doctor should give you advice on the best doses for you according to your condition.

Doses also present a major challenge because herbs have properties depending on seasons, climate, soil, altitude, time of the day when they are collected, and the environment in general. If you cook with herbs and grow Mediterranean herbs in North American cold regions, you may have noticed you need larger amounts of your cultivated herbs than the amounts you would use if you buy herbs imported from Mediterranean countries. The same applies to herbs used in therapies. Only extensive practice with herbs will guide you to determine the right doses. Unfortunately issues attached to doses for herbs are not common knowledge in North America because western science does not understand use of herbs.

Supplements decreasing pain

The following table describes the top supplements for pain relief.

Names	Benefits
Antioxidants and multivitamins	To protect you from deficiencies, such as pain and inflammation, weakening the body. • Vitamin A protects brain cells • Vitamin C manufactures neurotransmitters and protects the brain from free radicals • Vitamin E slows the aging of the brain • B-complex vitamins promote proper functioning of the nervous system • Vitamin B2 reduces migraine, vitamin B6 reduces carpal tunnel syndrome, TMJ disorder and back pain; in addition, it increases pain resistance.
Boswellin	To reduce the number of white blood cells moving to inflamed areas
Bromelain	To provide an anti-inflammatory effect
Calcium	To relax muscle tissue and, as well as vitamin D, to prevent migraines
Capsaicin (the hot ingredient found in chili peppers)	To deplete substance P used by nerve cells to send pain signals. Capsaicin can be taken as food, in a capsule, or applied topically.
Devil's claw	To relieve pain and inflammation
Enzymes	To digest proteins to be obtained from a health store
Feverfew	To reduce migraine frequency
Fish oil	To reduce inflammation
Gamma-linolenic acid (GLA)	To provide anti-inflammatory properties
Ginger	To reduce inflammation in musculoskeletal disorders, to reduce nausea, blocking histamine, to decrease the number of bad prostaglandins, to prevent or treat migraines
Ginkgo biloba	To improve cerebral circulation
Ginseng	To give energy without nervous tension
Glucosamine and chondroitin	To build up new tissues and to reduce osteoarthritis
Kava	To reduce anxiety and muscle tension

Magnesium	To relax muscles, to calm nerves, to reduce migraines even if we do not know exactly why it works
Niacinamide and quercetin	To ease pain of osteoarthritis
Phenylalanine	To help stop the breakdown of endorphins
St. John's wort	To use as an antidepressant. An oil extract of this plant serves as an anti-inflammatory
Turmeric	To help as an anti-inflammatory and to provide an ingredient, curcumin, as powerful as cortisone and ibuprofen
Valerian	To sleep better and relax muscle
White willow	To relieve inflammation and pain.[57]

You should never take these supplements without discussing them with your physicians because these products can interact with medication and because you will need directions for suggested doses. Some of the above products are plants but herbs are not safe to use without control; just think that numerous powerful poisons come from plant.

Feverfew is a wild flower growing well in the Balkans and looking like daisies, used by ancient Greeks to treat fever and many other conditions, which reemerged about two thousand years later in the late 1970s in Britain to treat migraine. This herb would eliminate about one-fourth of all headaches, has no apparent ill effects and is sold in health food stores.[58] No promotion is made because the plant does not bring much money: patents are impossible to get on a plant and patented products bring money. For this reason more revenues can be made from prescription medications than from plants.[59]

Since no major revenue can be made, scientific research, sponsored by pharmaceutical companies looking for revenues, does not pay much attention to this flower. Ginger would have been used in Asia for centuries and is also, just like feverfew, a plant ignored by science apparently for financial reasons. Feverfew and ginger are good examples of the way businesses control products available to manage pain.

So, to summarize, think green and eat leafy vegetables such as kale, broccoli, spinach and chard which are loaded with B-complex vitamins, with chemicals encouraging the production of serotonin, and with magnesium which helps relax muscles.[60] Eat beans which are loaded with calcium and magnesium and prevent or treat migraines.[61] Fresh food is also full of L-tryptophan. Avoid pro-inflammatory fats such as butter, corn oil, full-fat dairy products – frozen non fat yogurt is much better than regular ice cream -, margarine, shortening and red meat; prefer to eat olive oil, salmon, tuna, sardines, pumpkin seeds, walnuts, dried figs, whole grains high in magnesium and having more nutrients than white bread, and rice which are also pain-safe foods.[62] Drink water and avoid also common fast fried food for another reason: it will increase your weight and will force your joints to work more!

CONCLUSION

The magic of all this? If you find manipulating vitamins and nutrients too complicated, the only starting action is to ask a therapist, if possible a dietician, to draft you a few menus and give you basic information. Another alternative is to purchase a book on the Mediterranean diet which remains one of the best in the world. The nature of this diet, loaded with antioxidants from fruits and vegetables controlling pain, is probably the reason why nutritional books, vitamins and supplements are not big sellers in the Mediterranean countries.

The rest may come as if by magic: if you are sure to do the best for your body, your mind will heal you and manage all your needs attached to serotonin and other substances which are not a worry at all on the shore of the Mediterranean sea. Your body is able to create the main chemicals needed to feed the brain. So only a few things are required of you: relax, have fruits and vegetables each day, eat fresh food prepared with love, avoid animal fat or added fat in fried food, have faith and trust the process just like a good friend! All the rest will come by itself.

This section on nutrition is intended to give you ideas and suggest a few nutrients to explore. In this area also you make choices and decide to follow the ones that work best for you. You are unique and food, just like medications, does not have the same effect on everybody. Coffee can give or prevent migraines. I find coffee very relaxing because it forces me to calm down and a hot drink always leaves me feeling good. Caffeine is said to have analgesic powers that can be used to fight headaches and is often added to aspirin, acetaminophen, and ibuprofen to enhance their effects. Caffeine's painkilling action may suppress our natural defenses to pain[63] but more research seems to be necessary to understand better why foods have totally different impacts on different people. Debates on food tend to be influenced by cultural beliefs. Caffeine is said to increase intelligence among school children in Italy, while in Northern America it is perceived as a substance that depletes calcium in the body. Of course vitamin D maintaining calcium in the body and obtained from sun exposure on the skin is not an issue in Italy. People with chronic pain need calcium to maintain the body in top shape and anything, such as coffee, threatening calcium becomes more of an issue in Northern America than it is in sunnier places.

Chocolate is another controversial food. It gives me comfort and relaxes me; but for others, chocolate possibly triggers migraines because of its cruel chemical ability to encourage inflammation.[64] All in all, nutrition is a personal matter.

Last word on these essential physical therapies

In conclusion, I would like to share a few essential components of physical therapy that I learned in my nine years of varied therapeutic interventions and visits to expensive health centres. The relationship between client and caregiver is as important as (and maybe more important than) any physical therapy provided. Physical therapy has an impact on the body but the natural painkillers in the nervous system are activated by the mind; physical therapy is aimed at developing these painkillers; if the mind sends a message of non-compatibility or danger to the client, the number of natural painkillers will not increase and pain will persist. In my experience if the client and the therapist get along well and if the relationship is good, subconscious processes within the client will seek to please the therapist and create success. It means the client's subconscious mind will "order" the natural painkillers to develop to ensure that physical therapy succeeds. So, this means that even if you can't afford expensive memberships in health clubs, even if you dream with your feet in the bathtub instead of visiting fancy spas, even if you get massages from someone who is not certified, you will heal if you manage to establish a positive relationship with your caregiver. Physical therapy is not about suffering in a gym and sweating on machines, it is about encouraging the painkillers in your nervous system to develop by bonding with caregivers.

On the other hand, you are responsible for taking charge of your health and ensuring your natural painkilling substances work. Nutrition helps but the reality of good nutrition is as cultural as it is scientific. Here I do not mean that your injuries are non-existent, indeed, your injuries can be catastrophic. I do not mean you do not get better because you consciously decided to remain unwell. I should add that therapists who failed to evoke a change in my physical condition, often accused me of being responsible for my failures and insisted their treatments were excellent in spite of my lack of response. Here I mean that the physical therapists are teachers. They do not work on you, they work with you, how ever catastrophic your injuries may be. You learn from them what is good for you and you practice it as long as your mind works.

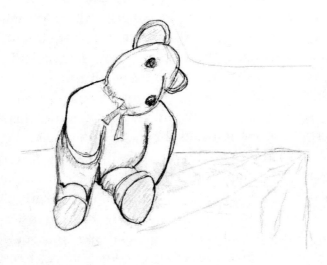

Chapter 4

PSYCHOLOGY

EARLY MORNING ROUTINE

6 o'clock am. October. Alarm clock ringing. Dark outside. Maybe raining? Stretch legs and arms to wake up muscles. Use hands to get up from bed and stop alarm. Cold. More stretches. Exercises to turn head to the right and the left. Neck stuck as usual. Headaches. Vague nausea. Take medication. Use stairs to go down to the kitchen. Still cold and dizzy. Make coffee very slowly. Find a cup which is not too heavy to hold. A bit sad. Take coffee cup to living room. Sit on chesterfield to rest head. More stretches. Try to smile. Get the blood flow running in the shoulders and arms. Have coffee. Cup heavy. Medication kicking in.

Daylight coming. Headache. Worried about upcoming hours. Too busy at work. Position in jeopardy? Someone alleged medical appointments affected performance. Doctors say this issue is political. Need to work to pay the bills. Maybe appointment with chiropractor after work should be cancelled. Too late anyway. Will cancel massage therapy next week if pain decreases.

NoV. 6, 2007

Really hard to breathe. Rib out of place in the back? Impossible to reach with the hand. Muscle spasms in the neck and shoulders. Muscle knots on shoulders make it difficult to hold cup. Time to move and get ready to work. Must keep working to pay for medical bills. 7:00 am. Time to wake up children. Still cold. Raise temperature in the house. Find a sweater. Too much pain in jaws to eat breakfast. Go upstairs. Wake the children. Hug them. Kiss them. Put lights on in their bedrooms. Turn on radio in their rooms to give them music. Waking up must be a pleasant experience for them. More kisses.

Have hot shower while kids have breakfast. Plug bathtub to save water to soak shoulders and neck in water. More stretches in bath water. More flexibility in the neck. Great news! It will be possible to drive to work! Make up session. Hide marks under the eyes. Lots of pink on cheeks to look healthy. Find a cheerful dress to compensate for puffy eyes. After all, the essential is invisible, said St-Exupery, so it is OK to cover up pain with make up. Very sad.

Worried pain will be there for rest of life. How to find a solution? Get dressed. Call one daughter to get her help to zip up pretty orange dress. Tell kids to get dressed really quickly. As usual, running late. Feel bad about telling kids to rush. 8:00 am. Can't move quickly. Still very stiff. Nausea. Pain in the neck. Unable to carry kids' backpacks to car. Kids grab their lunch boxes and school bags. We leave the house. Hard to back up van on the driveway (this neck does not want to collaborate!). Drop off kids in the home of a mom living near the school. Blow kisses from the car to children. Drops of rain on the windshield. Drops of tears on the face. Of course no reason to cry. Maybe sad because pain is still there even with medication. Guess it is OK to cry because kids do not see it. Try to smile in the rear view mirror. Wonderful waterproof mascara! Fifteen minutes fighting rush hour traffic. Practice smiling to look dynamic and professional at work.

This was my early morning story for years. It is not unique and I share it with a large number of people experiencing chronic pain. What to do? My TMJ specialist, who heard my story, sent me to a psychologist. That was an excellent idea. Pain is an emotional "response" to an injury and usually causes suffering. Quite often this suffering erodes energy, which is the source of life, and prevents it from flowing freely in the body.

Psychologists deal with this suffering component and reduce it.

Most physicians are scientists who like singular cause-and-effect relationships. However "almost all chronic, degenerative conditions have multiple causes, and require multiple therapies."[1] One of these therapies is psychological.

> **Without undergoing a winter that bites into your bones How can the plum blossoms regale you With their piercing fragrance?**
>
> Huang Po cited by Bedard, 1999, p. 36.

Psychotherapy is very important since chronic pain always has a major mental component and is managed by the brain.[2] Psychotherapy allows personal development, forces you to examine your life, energizes the body, and restores minds which are able to become at peace with pain. This does not mean that pain disappears for ever; it means that we accept pain and organize our lives with a pain component. However suffering will decrease and consequently, pain will also decrease. Being at peace with pain will offer you this type of healing.

NEED FOR KIND SUPPORT

Psychotherapy may help you to change the conditions of your life because pain decreases when we are surrounded with kindness and support. On the other hand, pain increases when we are in a toxic environment or in a toxic relationship. Yes, pain is highly negotiable and loaded with fluctuations. It helps to be in the right place and in the right family to heal. In 1854, the Lady of the Lamp, Florence Nightingale, cared for injured soldiers in the Crimean War. In so doing, she founded universal care and modern nursing. She believed you did not "fix people; you try to create the conditions that will allow them to heal themselves."[3] People living with chronic pain need a space to accept this pain and heal.

If pain does not disappear because of the nature of our physical issues and because we are not in the right environment with the right relationships, even if psychotherapy is unable to change our conditions of life, psychotherapy will give us tools to transform our pain into something life-enhancing. Energy spent on fighting pain can be directed to

> *Each look, each movement, every word and tone*
> *Should tell your patient you are all his own;*
> *Not the mere artist, purchased to attend,*
> *But the warm, ready, self-forgetting friend*
> *Whose genial visit in itself combines*
> *The best of cordials, tonics, anodynes.*
>
> A 19th century poem by Oliver Wendell Holmes using Florence Nightingale's ideas and defining a healing relationship between client and caregiver.[4]

JUNE 18, 2017 LAST

another purpose, such as helping others or volunteering for a great cause.

THE SECRET OF PSYCHOLOGICAL CARE

Why do people make an appointment with a psychologist? Quite often they arrange a visit without knowing what a psychologist could do for them. They make an appointment because they were asked to see a psychologist by one of their other caregivers who perhaps had exhausted other ways to deal with the pain issue; or they arrange a visit because they are depressed or are looking for someone to hear their complaints. Do you remember hearing *"only crazy people see a psychologist"* or the pejorative meaning to *"pain is all in the mind"?* Because our society takes a negative view of those who visit psychologists, clients do not openly discuss their visits to a psychologist. Many others who work in business and handle money, who are in the field of transportation, who manage people or look after children, do not even consider getting help from a psychologist; they do not look for help by fear of these appointments becoming known to others and by fear of possible loss of employment as a consequence. Unfortunately society associates psychotherapy with mental illness, and mental illness with danger. The impact of these irrational societal attitudes is called "stigma."

Most people are unaware of what a psychologist can do to help control chronic pain. I should add here I noticed young children and teenagers know a few accurate facts about psychologists because schools often call on these therapists to act as counselors for the students. My 13 year-old daughter used to call them "the doctors who cure bad thoughts in the mind" and at this age children do not see any stigma in talking to one of them. Attitudes towards psychologists appear to change later on in life.

So what can psychologists offer? They put their clients back on the right track. They can help prevent pain from taking over lives; they reassure us and assist our exploration of our subconscious processes; they teach how to make the mind stronger and use it in order to reduce pain. They can help to change negative attitudes; they suggest tools for coping and promote healing on the physical, mental and spiritual levels. Most of them really care for you (even if they are not allowed to show it to you for ethical reasons). They can also improve your quality of life by suggesting changes to get away from a toxic job or toxic relationships that make it more difficult to be at peace with pain. However only the clients can choose to allow a psychologist to make a difference in their life because clients are the ones who must learn how to control pain and work to change their perceptions. If you choose to include psychotherapy in your quest to find peace with pain, you *ipso facto* decide to take decisive action by yourself without relying solely on medication and doctors, and without leaving the solution to therapists. In psychotherapy, there is no best technique and there is no magic formula to develop inner strength. The following approaches, promoting integrative medicine and making space for spirituality, give good results and are compatible. They all require will and practice. However the mind is not known to have narrow limits, and possibilities of healing through the mind are essentially endless.

ATTITUDE TO HEAL LIFE

Attitude means a psychological characteristic, belief, or posture, usually adopted without reflection. Cultural and family beliefs have an impact on attitude[5] and may make it difficult to change attitudes. However attitudes should be modified when they are negative and when they affect the body making acceptance or adaptation to pain impossible. So, one does well to heal one's life before attempting to heal one's chronic pain. Inherent in healing a broken life is the promise of acceptance and recovery from pain.

Excellence or perfection?

Perfectionism is one of the most important attitudinal imperfections affecting recovery from chronic pain. Perfectionism can be an illness and a type of obsession. The shift is in priorities inherent in abandoning the road to perfection. It can be a blessing for your health. It is healthy to seek excellence; it is unhealthy to seek perfection because perfection does not exist and cannot be achieved. This implies doing laundry less often or cleaning the oven less often. It also implies ignoring any negative comments from people around you if you drop everything and go out for a walk. One does well to place one's own needs first as much as possible, and to do what feels good. Negative thoughts can be changed by interrupting them and developing positive alternatives.[6]

Of course dealing with pain takes time, and any activity requires additional energy when we are in pain. Target specific elements in your attitude that you would like to improve or change. It can be difficult to modify thoughts affecting attitudes and to abandon the habit of catastrophizing because pain distorts thinking. Adaptation is necessary and we must believe we are very valuable human beings even if we are in pain. As it was explained to me by one of my psychologists, people are just like lamps. They come in different sizes, different shapes, different colors. However all have a light inside. We should believe that we are all valuable and hold a light in spite of chronic pain. Positive attitudes will change the perception of pain and will change the way we act. This will reduce suffering in the same manner as hopelessness and depression increase it.[7]

Coping skills

Behavioral therapists try to stop self-destructive behaviors without uncovering a deep neurotic cause. Chronic pain can cause many negative behaviors, such as having no social life, and behavior therapists attempt to intervene at the level of the destructive activities themselves, replacing them by new coping strategies. Commonly recommended coping skills include distractions (such as going out), asking for help and introducing positive elements in your life (such as relaxation).[8] These help to direct the attention away from pain and encourage a non-attachment to any felt pain.

Replacing old habits with newly-mastered skills takes time and discipline. I know from personal experience it is extremely hard for mothers with young children to put personal needs first and to accept imperfection. However changing attitude and taking morphine have at least one common attribute: both help to decrease pain by facilitating enjoyment in life. They do not act directly on the pain, rather they develop pleasure in life. Both have an impact on the brain. Pain and pleasure are closely related brain functions. Endorphins help to fight pain as well as to create comfort. Laughing and positive attitudes heal because pleasure, just like pain, travels in the body.[9] If we change our attitudes, we are able to find greater enjoyment in ordinary experiences such as a beautiful sunset or sunrise, flowers, rainbows, smiles, a symphony, a photo, friends or hugs. Beauty is essential. As we all know, seeing something sad evokes sad feelings. Seeing beauty and presenting a good image of ourselves make us feel good. Have you noticed how suffering disappears and pain decreases when we are at the lake, connect with nature, watch the sea, or look at the mountains?

Natural tools

There is a hidden reason explaining why the mind is so powerful in its effects on chronic pain. This reason is that chronic pain does not travel fast. "The nervous system's transmission of pain is inefficient."[10] Chronic pain crawls along neurons at three miles per hour while other nerve signals, including the touch signals, travel at 200 miles per hour. Because of their slow speed, "the signals of chronic pain can be thwarted by crowding the brain with competing sources of input," including positive thoughts.[11] These calm thoughts also decrease pain by forcing the body to "secrete chemicals that block pain."[12] These pain-killing chemicals include the endorphins released by the neurotransmitters, present in large quantities and coming from the mind-power effect.[13]

Optimism, empathy and altruism towards others are also great tools when facing pain. Optimism shows us we are in control of our life even if there is uncertainty around us. It prevents depression and allows us to see a light at the end of the tunnel. If we concentrate on others, we focus less on our own pain. Psychotherapy teaches us how to anticipate pleasant experiences and maintain positive thoughts. It trains us to stop evaluating and assessing our feelings and activities; it allows us to see the importance of being connected with others and of understanding other's needs. Of course this is not easy when we are in pain and it takes time to change attitudes. Determination will help you to go through the wall of pain and produce natural substances that decrease pain. Marathon runners often face this wall of pain and complete the race because of their determination; their pain decreases at the point of arrival.[14]

AFFIRMATIONS TO BRING COMFORT

Affirmations are short positive statements or quotes to repeat to ourselves when we need comfort.[15] They are similar to brainwashing but at the same time they can be life savers! Repeating them several times per day strengthens the newer positive attitude they imply.[16] Repetition also creates a belief thus having a strong impact on pain, energy, actions and emotions. Of course when we do an affirmation, we must have a sincere desire to change in order to see a benefit. We can make affirmations on our own when we are in a challenging position and they can give us the energy to continue. "I am finding peace" and "My mind is in control" are two of my preferred affirmations helping me to cope. You could develop your own affirmations. The mind-power effect is "a force that literally puts mind over matter" and decreases the pain.[17] Visualization is another highly effective technique to reach a positive mind-power response.[18]

LAUGHTER TO REACH PEACE

What about laughing as a therapy? Yes, I am serious. Of course it takes time to learn how to laugh when we are in pain. My 13 year-old daughter has a wonderful explanation. She explained that I did not laugh very much because I am tired and consequently my lips are unable to curl up any more. A great logical interpretation by a little girl! Fortunately when I am in the right space, surrounded by the ones who care about me, I manage to laugh. Just like other relaxation techniques, laughing requires practice.

> We don't laugh because we are happy. We are happy because we laugh.
> Williams James cited by Cobb, 1996, p.113.

Laughter is a wonderful ally in the quest for peace with pain; it heals because of its physical, psychological and spiritual components. It helps us to digest and to sleep. However first of all, laughter reduces stress that very easily prevents recovery from chronic pain. In addition stress lowers the pain threshold. Stress also causes headaches and high blood pressure, damages the stomach, causes strokes, disturbs the rhythm of the heartbeat, lowers levels of white blood cells and weakens the immune system. Stress is defined as a physiological reaction to a perceived danger. Because it is linked to a perception and to a reaction, stress does not have the same impact on everyone. It is possible to change our perceptions, learn to laugh and to relax in order to modify our reactions to stressors.

A good workout

Chronic pain and issues attached to family, money and work are major causes of stress. Sometimes it is more difficult to understand reasons causing muscular tension and stress. Accidental injury may make impossible a lifestyle that once seemed reasonable. Emotions, small issues at work or in the family, and other minor stressors such as heat or cold can then cause enormous pain. As a consequence, relaxation becomes essential.

Deep breathing is a quick and efficient way to decrease stress even if we do not know the reasons for a specific stressful condition. Laughing is also an excellent technique to fight stress and decrease pain. How does it work? Laughter moves the muscles on the face, the abdomen, the diaphragm, the ribs, the shoulders and arms; and it has a significant impact on the heart beat, arteries, blood pressure and …. lungs! You see, laughter empties lungs by rejecting toxins together with a very large amount of air, and laughter pushes exhaling to the highest maximum beyond control by lungs elasticity. A good laugh gives the same sensations as a workout.

Laughter cleans up the body, decreases stress, inflammation and muscle tension on a long term basis, it can take us to a sort of "high" and becomes an analgesic by increasing the number of our little friends, the endorphins. At the same time we develop resistance to stressors without being forced to eliminate the ones common in a normal life. Of course laughter offers distractions and can make it sometimes impossible to feel pain! Finally laughter helps us remain positive and enjoy life even if many days can be tough.[19]

SENSES TO ENJOY BEAUTY

Activities attached to senses are great healers, especially if they hold a beauty component. Touching and being touched physically are essential for healing. Heat and massages can give an extraordinary feeling of well-being. Hot showers, saunas and towels warmed up in a dryer are of high benefit to decrease several forms of pain, even if they have no positive impact on sunburn pain (also called neuropathic pain). Mental warmth, expressed by touching and confirming friendship, love and intimacy, is very important in healing. To be held and hugged by another caring person is one of the best ways to fight pain. Seeing provides another excellent tool. We all know that light heals and decreases depression. Similarly, peaceful and sunny landscapes, even on photos, also heal. A form of healing meditation is based on hearing relaxing music and visualizing parts of the body surrounded by appropriate colors. The lower part of the spine is seen in red, the navel in orange, the solar plexus in yellow, the heart in green, the throat in blue, the front head in purple, the area above the head in transparent crystal. This exercise follows the seven centers of physical, psychological and spiritual energy called *chakras* by Oriental cultures.

Music as a magical treatment

Hearing is another important sense in healing pain. Music is noted to develop the immune system and endorphins, the

> It is looking at things for a long time that ripens you and gives you a deeper understanding.
>
> Painter Vincent Van Gogh cited by George, 2000, p. 94.

natural painkillers in the brain, because of the chemical reactions coming from rich emotions and joy born from music. Of course music decreases negative feelings. Have you noticed how many dentists use music in their offices? Music promotes synchrony of the brain waves, a phenomenon that also happens during relaxation. Music changes the body temperature and has a positive impact on our adaptation to changes in hot and cold temperatures. It improves breathing by decreasing or increasing its speed before finding the right balance. Music also has an impact on heart beat, blood pressure and is even said to make learning easier. It develops memory and may even make people more intelligent. Students get higher marks when they are exposed to music. Other benefits attributed to music include decreased stress, increased productivity and endurance, and improved digestion and security.

Music also allows communication and sharing of emotions, reflections of good memories, and the sort of freedom of emotions that is common among children. Music helps to develop a sense of belonging to a group and facilitates interpersonal relationships. Numerous articles have been written on the healing impact of music on illnesses, such as cancer, autism, paralysis and schizophrenia.

Wellness from smell and taste

The chemical senses are important. Pleasant smells (such as the ones from a cake or from flowers) allow a connection with something good; these smells have a positive impact on the brain and can decrease pain. Aromatherapy, which is discussed in another chapter, is said to heal, but unfortunately few comprehensive studies on aromatherapy have been published. There are two important reasons for this lack. First, it is difficult to present smells and tastes as stimuli in a controlled fashion. Second, smells and tastes are complex and do not lend themselves readily to the reductionism inherent in western science. Smell and taste are connected. Several scientific studies have been conducted on the link between food and bioavailability of neurotransmitters, such as serotonin and endorphins, both of which have been implicated in relief of pain. Comfort food is not a myth! Certain types of food have an impact on the chemical messengers in the brain, modifying our emotions and appetite. Hot pepper protects from pain by eliminating a chemical called "P substance" found in the nerve cells. This substance allows the sensory cells to communicate pain to the brain. It is very simple: if there is no "P substance", the cells cannot transmit pain information. Hot pepper is not bad for you and certainly easier for the stomach than many anti-inflammatory medications. Another chapter will provide detailed information on food recommended to decrease pain. Personally chocolate gives me a feeling of well-being, and I find a meal with spicy food really brings a good dose of comfort, especially if shared with friends and family.[20]

MIND-BODY APPROACH TO HEAL WITHIN AND BETWEEN PERSONS

Pain begins as a physical signal but quickly takes on psychological and interpersonal dimensions.[21] Pain management is a "mind game"[22] even if most people in our western culture do not like the idea of mitigating pain through psychotherapy. Asian cultures tend to be willing to join mind and body. In fact, the Chinese word for "mind" is the same as the word for "heart". In contrast, North American medical specialties are defined according to organs and organ "systems". Our culture makes a clear distinction between physicians looking after the body and psychologists or psychiatrists responsible for the mind. However we know this division is artificial because emotions have an obvious impact on the body, and vice-versa. When you laugh, are happy, mix with loving and caring people supporting you, pain abates. When you are busy reading a book or are distracted by something you like, it is possible to forget or ignore pain. So the mind-body is more than a link. It is an identity: mind and body are one, and dividing them for the sake of discussion is of questionable merit, especially with respect to the topic of pain and comfort. Unfortunately the term "psychosomatic illness", which means disease caused in the body by the mind, has a very bad interpretation amongst lay persons in our society. It is a real stigma because the understanding is: the brain causes the disease, the disease is not real. This meaning is taken as confluent with mental illness. Of course, mental disease is not well perceived in our world where everybody competes for excellence.

However the contrary is also possible. The brain can have a positive impact on the body. Just smile! Close your eyes and see your pain leaving you with the help of pink hot air balloons! Watch nasty people around you slowly fading and replace them by loving ones! Open your eyes! Most probably, and I hope it is the case, you feel better just by reading these lines. I confess I feel more relaxed by only writing these suggestions. One of us has practiced the zen meditation of simply sitting and grinning for 10-15 minutes upon awakening. The impact of this simple process completely banished a major depressive episode in less than one week. Yes, breathing, meditation, and hypnosis help your mind to reduce chronic pain which can be seen as "adverse chronic stress" because pain as well as a chronically stressed state destroy our balance by causing the exhaustion of recuperative abilities.[23] These mental therapies also help you to enjoy life even if you are in pain.

Biofeedback was developed to provide a visual or sound description of the level of tension in the various parts of the body. Relaxation techniques can be combined to reduce muscle tension and, as a consequence, pain. Tension causes migraines and headaches, muscle knots and spasms... in other words, tension causes pain. When tension settles in injured parts of the body, pain increases; it becomes useful to reduce tension (or relax) in order to reduce pain. Relaxation techniques relieve muscle spasms, release endorphins to relieve pain and also help you to gain control of the pain experience.[24] In addition, people who use these techniques gain a sense of mastery no medication can ever provide. These techniques are gaining credibility among physicians, but most books about chronic pain, written by medical doctors, overlook the mind-body approach. Thus, this therapy remains unknown to the majority of physicians providing chronic pain therapy.[25]

The power of the mind

The mind is seen as "a major factor in healing within the single person" but also is "a factor in healing both within and between persons."[26] This chapter treats therapies of the mind and includes "any therapy in which effects of consciousness bridge between different persons."[27] You will find, in the type of universal and infinite mental therapy, forms of distance healing reached through intercessory prayers, compassionate thoughts or intentions and through imagery created by one person for the benefit of another one in pain.[28] The whole of transpersonal psychology deals in this domain. These distance healing therapies work better when people are connected and share the same beliefs because they are based on faith and intuition. The focus is on mind rather than brain. Reported phenomena include miracle cures. Only recently have they been considered as apt topics for scientific research projects. These phenomena are beginning to be mentioned at the university level in medical schools holding sessions on spirituality, and it is likely they will receive more attention in future years.

I like this concept of eternity medicine because it brings the feeling of never being alone or lonely even when I am physically by myself. The experience of immaterial ongoing support coming from distant loving persons helps one negotiate pain flares and is invaluable for managing depression. Non local therapies are compatible with more traditional mental therapies whose effectiveness is improved in an atmosphere of belief that we are loved by others and we are a part of a loving universe. People who have no such belief do not do as well, as people who do, even with traditional therapies.

We will concentrate on mental strategies helping to control the body and to reduce several physical issues within the person. This is called the "mind-body interaction."[29] The mind and the body must be trained to manage pain and function together. No results come quickly, and if I have little time to relax, I find medication to be very effective. As you may suspect, we believe mental strategies and medication should work together and are both valid parts of pain control and management.

BREATHWORK TO ENTER AN ALTERED STATE

We are not trained to breathe properly from the diaphragm and we tend to breathe silently from the chest. Women tend to breathe the most from the upper part of the chest. I realized this when I entered into the world of chronic pain. Breathing while in pain was very difficult. It took two pain specialists to teach me how to place my hand on the abdomen and raise it slowly while breathing deeply before exhaling slowly. This simple technique decreases muscle tension. It is invaluable to practice at work, under stress, to manage pain flares, or to fall nicely asleep.

I prefer to breathe deeply while lying on my back, but it is possible to do it in any position. Similar breathing techniques, called *pranayama* in Sanskrit, are used in yoga and during zen meditations (zen is a Japanese word, *chan* is the Chinese equivalent). It is interesting to note that in our modern western culture, women are trained to be elegant and maintain a flat abdomen and in the past, they were forced to wear rigid tops.[30] This posture together with fashionable narrow clothes has added to the social convention of not making noise with the body. It is impossible to maintain such conventions during deep breathing requiring the abdomen to move in and out. This type of breathing is also called "diaphragmatic" because the diaphragm contracts at the beginning of each breath, when the abdominal wall moves out when air is pulled into the lungs. When the diaphragm relaxes, the breath moves out and the abdomen flattens or even sinks.[31]

Our need for the constituents of air is arguably the most pressing biological need we have of our environment. We can do without food for about 30 days; without water, for three days or so. Without air we die within minutes. Every meditative method in the world attends to the breath. Every relaxation strategy attends to the breath. This is because attending to the breath provides the most direct means of influencing the energy flow of the body.

Breathing for healing

Breathwork is a powerful method of promoting personal growth and awareness. It can be used therapeutically (to treat various disorders and symptoms) and as a meditative strategy. Of course breathwork is spiritual by definition. The word "inspiration" means both to breathe and to be uplifted in spirit. Formal breathwork utilizes conscious controlled breathing methods to induce an altered state in which insight and personal growth is facilitated. As you surrender to the rhythm of your breathing, the conscious intellect releases, and you gain more direct access to subconscious powers, processes and materials.

A major advantage of the kind of altered state induced by breathwork is that you achieve deep relaxation after a few minutes of breathwork and, if needed, return to normal consciousness within moments, simply by normalizing the breathing and by breathing less deeply. Breathwork can take you quickly to a safe altered state which is maintained through conscious control of the deep breathing. The experience of breathwork is transcendental. That means it is possible to experience yourself at several ages and/or places at once. Parallels and associations between (for example) physical symptoms, emotional issues, memories and mental attitudes are commonly clarified during breathwork.

If your close your eyes, if you do deep breathwork for a few minutes and let your mind wander, you may see yourself in your childhood. This is an altered state where age is transcended. It may be useful to remember your childhood, if chronic pain comes from a physical condition added to an unhappy childhood. Breathwork taking you to the past may allow you to see issues having an impact on your pain. It removes the defense system and helps us to regress and uncover these buried problems preventing healing and giving a meaning to our pain. When causes are identified, we can release them and remove a source aggravating physical pain. These issues should be shared with your psychologist who can provide counseling on the best way to treat problems that have a negative impact on your physical condition and exacerbate pain. Healing becomes transformation and personal development. The client coached by a psychologist is responsible for the change and for recovery.

Deep breathing can be combined with visualization to become even more effective. In order to focus when bombarded with thousands of thoughts, I like to imagine air coming in through my mouth and leaving from my navel, forming a complete circle. However the most efficient visualization for me is to imagine my garden in full bloom. I do an imaginary journey, starting from one end of the garden and usually pain disappears or sleep comes in before I reach the other end of my garden. Breathing takes place in front of each flower and, in my imaginary visit, I concentrate on the scent and shape of the flowers. When I am unable to sleep and get rid of heavy thoughts, I simply breathe deeply for a few minutes and I fall asleep. Just try it! There are no side effects, and it is free.

Breathing can also reduce suffering by helping to acknowledge pain rather than being upset and fighting against spasms and trigger points. Deep breathing helps to relieve suffering if we acknowledge we hurt and if we keep breathing in spite of this pain. Breathwork is of high interest because it can be done anywhere, even in public places if done with discretion. You inhale from the nose and exhale from the nose or the mouth. Exhaling from the nose tends to induce sleep, so it is recommended to exhale from the mouth during daily activities. About ten breaths are enough to relax and decrease pain.

Why is breathing so quick and effective at decreasing pain? Diaphragmatic breathing "helps shift brain waves away from the excitatory beta brain-wave frequency to the calming alpha frequency."[32] Intense pain takes place when the brain operates in the beta-wave frequency. Breathing also supplies oxygen and removes carbon dioxide from the cells, regulates the body's acidity and alkalinity, and helps the elimination of water, hydrogen, methane and other toxins. Lack of this elimination increases inflammation and sensitizes nerves.[33]

MEDITATION, VISUALIZATION, AND CONTEMPLATION to heal faster

Meditation may be described as the spirituality of being aware of your surroundings and your inner world.[34] It brings peace of mind and awareness by removing thoughts from the mind. It allows you to understand what is buried inside you and also to have a better idea of what is important in life. It recharges and revitalizes mind and body, increases the production of serotonin in the brain and draws the electrical activities of the

> *Beauty and joy, however, can be experienced in the most industrial of landscapes or the most difficult living situations. Meditation is a good way of taking time out and allowing yourself to tune into and appreciate the moment, whether you happen to be walking along the seashore, sitting by a stream, or just noticing and enjoying the intensity of silence in a still room.*
>
> Hudson, 2003, p. 6.

brain into an alpha state similar to light sleep. It lowers blood pressure and develops antibodies. It trains you to focus, and reduces stress, depression and anxiety.[35] Meditation provides an opportunity to think about issues and visualize solutions leading to healing and happiness. The light of truth and knowledge is called awareness or enlightenment. Obviously everyone can benefit from meditation because it trains one to analyze actions, observe, develop insight, find a balance, be sensitive to others, be compassionate, be loving, and mindful all the time, and to heal. This is the nature of awareness or enlightenment. It does not necessarily involve sectarian beliefs although meditation and Buddhism share the same goal. Several religions also use a form of meditation as a way to access a superior force. Meditation simply invites you to slow down and concentrate on something. This focus can be the repetition of a word (called *mantra*) silently or aloud, or of an idea, sound or a short sentence, leading to a feeling of wellbeing. The focus includes often concentrating on a color. The most common *mantra* in any languages is "om" found also in words such as *shalom, omen,* or *amen.* You can also focus your eyes on something pleasant and relaxing or listen to music. Colors hold messages. Red means energy, green, harmony, blue, peace, violet, beauty and dignity.[37] You can imagine the energy flowing freely through the *chakras.* However, the most common object for meditative focus is the breath. You need about 20 mn, once or twice a day, to meditate. When your mind is relaxed, your body is also relaxed. You do not have to buy expensive equipment to meditate.

Meditation is easy

How do you meditate? You sit in a relaxed position on the floor, on your heels or on a chair, in a peaceful and comfortable place without phones or distraction. You close your eyes, you concentrate and you breathe deeply at the same time. You remain passive throughout this meditation and gently send away any mental distraction coming to mind. Your sitting posture should be comfortable and it is said that sitting crossed-legged in the lotus position is best when you meditate. Sitting with a straight back is said to enhance the calming effects of meditation "since the nerves most critical to your overall well-being run up the spine."[38] You may place pillows under your knees to support your crossed legs and, if you wish, spray lavender, which has a calming effect, or burn sage or sweetgrass, or incense as a symbol of purification. When you close your eyes, you look inside yourself and find a focus bringing you peace and allowing you to relax.

I like a form of meditation including music and I find it very calming to visualize and imagine the colors and the perfumes attached to an image such as a flower or a garden. As usual, breathe deeply as soon as you close your eyes. There are no limits to the type of images supported by words: such as being in a very special place, walking by the sea or any other location found in nature, playing with children, listening to music, looking at the stars, imagining a beam of golden light dissolving pain or a healing light flowing through the body, are only a few examples of images. It is possible to practice meditation almost anywhere and even in public since no one can read your mind.

Repetition of ideas, verbally based and processed primarily in the left hemisphere of the brain, with images, processed primarily in the right hemisphere, is very powerful because it involves the entire brain.[39] In addition to changing perception, visualization, just like meditation, has a sedating effect and causes biochemical changes in the body. It stimulates the production of endorphins and calming neurotransmitters, such as serotonin, and it "reprograms the brain's cortex."[40] Visualization can be very healing in that it can be used to replace a negative image with a positive one. During visualization, "the more real you make your visualization, the more powerful will be its benefits."[41]

This means you can visualize yourself in excellent physical shape or see yourself as enjoying nature, especially since you should get some relief from this approach.

Meditation and visualization, which are easily combined, provide small breaks that can be taken during the day when muscle tension builds up and pain increases. Their effects can last for hours especially if different techniques, such as meditation, visualization and deep breathing are employed together. They are also very useful before falling asleep because you can keep night medication to a minimum. Another form of imagery is imagining a cool shower or a walk under the rain when inflammation of nerves causes sunburn pain to become very painful. It is better not to wait for this pain to increase too much, otherwise it tends to be more intense and takes more time to decrease. Personally I love connecting with nature. You may prefer to imagine you are standing on a bridge and to see you throwing your pain into the river; or you can see yourself on a train while you watch out the window and see your pain and worries going away in front of you. There is again no limit to this exercise.

Draw your pain

You can also give a shape and a color to your pain. The next step is to put your pain in a closed jar or see it dissolving in front of you. Another common exercise is to imagine a golden thread repairing injured tissues or to see your worries leaving the space around you. There are no limitations to the type of images putting a distance between you and your pain. It is possible to meditate and at the same time to lose concentration and have several thoughts coming at you. Please don't worry! When this happens, the best is to gently go back to the originally intended word, sound or image.

See your pain

Visualization presents the same advantage as meditation in that you can do it anywhere, at any time, when you are alone or in a crowd. It is your own interior and private world. No one else holds the key and you invite in whom you want and when you want, if you decide to include significant others. Visualization helps you to see decreasing pain or to stand in a painless world. Meditation and visualization, also called imagery, are priceless as therapies for chronic pain. They can be performed anywhere, they do not force you to do exhausting physical exercises, they are not expensive once you are able to practice them on your own and they really do help to decrease pain. It is then no surprise that pain can be seen as a sort of "mind game". However all these mental therapies involve diligent practice and willingness to invest time in mastering them. Athletes, artists, writers, and public speakers often use visualization as a form of rehearsal to be better prepared, relax before a public presentation and increase their chances of winning or doing well.

Visualization, like meditation, involves sitting or lying down in a calm and comfortable place, closing or fixating your eyes and relaxing while concentrating on an image. This can be a visual representation of a happy event or location, or it can be a visual symbol such as a red ball for damaged tissue. A symbol is less scary than the original injured tissue, therefore easier to visualize. You can also visualize an image of yourself in good health and physical condition. Visualization conditions the mind and also programs the body. As the brain conceives an act, it suggests that the body performs this action. I practice visualization where I see the muscles smooth and relaxed and as a consequence, my muscles do relax. It is also helpful to see fresh air coming into the mouth, the lungs and leaving the body through the navel in a circular movement. I like to reproduce this picture during breathwork in order to relax faster. Imagery works better if combined with meditation or hypnosis when the body is relaxed and works even better when combined with senses. If you see the colors of the flowers, smell the scents of the garden, feel the breeze on the skin, and hear the birds, imagery decreases pain even faster. Through the magic of visualization, mental pictures become a real physical visit to the garden.

Mindfulness

The entire metabolism changes with meditation as compared with resting. Less oxygen is consumed, less carbon dioxide is produced; breathing slows down; a very low level of a chemical lactate is found in the bloodstream and this indicates a deep peace. Brain wave patterns slow. Sometimes blood pressure goes down. This stress-reducing phenomenon is called the "relaxation response."[42] Stress reduction is important because tension can cause or complicate most (if not all) medical conditions. Relaxation decreases chronic pain, insomnia, anxiety, anger, and depression. Meditation sometimes gives an immediate feeling of well-being, but deep changes can take several weeks or months of practice.

I first noticed a change in the level of pain after a few sessions when all of a sudden I was aware that the pain was returning. I realized it had been absent for a few minutes without use of additional medication. When thoughts and feelings are observed, meditation can also lead to mindfulness which then increases a sense of connection with other people and the environment. Mindfulness does not only help to handle a health issue; it develops "a way of being" that may allow a greater appreciation of life. Of course this requires regular meditation and the will to be mindful in daily life.[43] Mindfulness helps to deepen insight, self-understanding and prevents one from reacting automatically to stress.[44] A meditative lifestyle is also consistent with the use of remote healing methods.

Contemplation is a sort of meditation involving visualization and deep breathing. You sit alone and quiet, in a peaceful place; for example, in a garden. If it is winter or if you have no access to a garden, you may place plants in a room, or create your own interior garden in your mind. Relaxing with deep breathing, you focus on a thought and study answers to a question or issue. This helps to develop ideas and solutions. If invading exterior thoughts come to your mind, you send them back calmly and you continue to focus on your first thought.

Work with your muscles!

Another form of meditation involves contracting and relaxing muscles from head to toes. We do not recommend this form of meditation or "progressive muscle relaxation" to the ones who already have tense muscles from pain. This could irritate injured muscles. We prefer another gentle method to communicate with muscles, and can concentrate on specific muscles, imagining they work well in a relaxed context. Unless you prefer to concentrate on specific muscles, you proceed from the forehead to the toes and visualize relaxed muscles in each part of the body. This mental exercise will decrease your pain. Relaxation is not easy for people having difficulty concentrating, for the ones who were physically active, for the ones experiencing traumatic events (such as a car collision or various forms of abuse), and for those who are simply worriers by nature. However if one takes the time to practice and gain mastery, anyone can learn relaxation techniques. Relaxation allows you to let worries, including pain, go away and teaches you to live for the moment without pain. It is essential to healing.

> The past is over, and you cannot be sure about the future, so the only time you can truly affect is now.
>
> Hudson, 2003, p. 54.

BIOFEEDBACK to be your mirror

Meditation and any other form of relaxation can be combined with biofeedback. Biofeedback is a technique similar to looking at yourself in a mirror, but instead of your exterior body, you deal with the interior of the body. Biofeedback is not a routine treatment recommended by many physicians. It was developed in the 1970s and can be slightly expensive. Despite decades of evidence supporting its clinical usefulness, biofeedback is not always funded by insurers. It is not painful and has no side effects, and involves using electronic instruments to provide an individual with an image or a sound that increases awareness of bodily processes and states. For the purpose of this discussion I am going to presume we are measuring muscle tension.

During a biofeedback session, you sit in a quiet and comfortable room. Electrical devices, called electrodes, are placed on the body. These are connected to a computer or a "black box" and reproduce on a monitor a pattern of lines or sounds giving feedback from our body indicating the level of muscle tension, temperature, skin resistance, and other measurable indicators. It measures small and invisible physiological changes in your body that would otherwise likely go unnoticed. The goal is to learn how to use the body and the brain to reduce the factors known to correlate with and/or contribute to discomfort. Biofeedback is also an approach providing you with an image or a sound that can in turn be used to control your state of well-being. Indicators employed in biofeedback include skin temperature, changes in perspiration, pulse rate and strength, respiration, and EEG frequency.[45] Therapy can target specific parts of the body where physical changes should be documented. Biofeedback is usually made available by psychologists as it bridges "the conscious and subconscious techniques"[46] because it involves the body and its control by the mind aiming at improving whatever parameter is being measured. It is a sort of mirror giving you a representation of physiological changes taking place in the body. When we are aware of these changes, it is easier to control them using the mind to relax the body. The client learns how it feels to be relaxed and it is then easier at a later time, without biofeedback, to reproduce the same feelings of relaxation. In addition, because it measures important parameters, biofeedback can provide objective data for insurance purposes.

The challenges of biofeedback

Biofeedback can be frustrating because of a few weaknesses associated with the system. First of all, it may be difficult to clearly identify the area which is tense, because only the client in pain is able to locate it using pain level. Pain is not a reliable indicator of muscle tension because compensation occurs and creates referred pain. Also pain can be found in perfectly healthy parts of the body, and may cause the therapist to place the sensor on incorrect parts of the body that are painful but otherwise uninvolved. The readings would then indicate false relaxation. Many times I told a massage therapist that my left elbow, wrist or front ribs were terribly painful, before stating my shoulders would be in perfect shape, only to discover two minutes later, when she touched my shoulders, that the neck and the shoulders were the primary source of the pain! Dysfunction in one part of the body often manifests itself as referred pain in another area of the body. Useful parameters for biofeedback are often not intuitively obvious (for example, the usefulness of hand temperature as a parameter for controlling migraine is not immediately obvious). A trained therapist may use foot reflexology to identify which part of the body is the main source of pain at the beginning of each visit. So many times I was wrong when I was asked where I had the most problems! Additionally it may take time to clearly identify the area to treat because one or two millimeters can be important in determining the level of pain. One area may feel normal until a finger touches this 1 mm spot and only then the problem area is identified.

The biofeedback system has also its own challenges. If

feedback is of muscle tension, the system peaks any time the muscles move, including during deep breathing, swallowing or talking. In real life it is almost impossible to maintain the low level of tension reported by the sensors during relaxed moments. It is also relatively easy to decrease the recorded tension, by slightly opening the mouth and especially by not moving muscles. This artificial posture is recorded as a relaxed position but it cannot be maintained over extended periods of time because it is not truly relaxed. On the other hand, when the machine indicates tension, it may be caused by muscle spasms which are almost impossible to control. Using the mind to decrease the spasms is very difficult in real life!

Add to this the fact that physical expression of any given psychological condition can manifest in more than one way. If you block expression through learned control of one parameter, the condition may manifest elsewhere.

Biofeedback can also be deceiving because the sensors monitor only a single parameter at one time, therefore people with multiple injuries may be forced to select sensor locations which are the most painful. As a consequence, the sensor can indicate the jaws or neck are relaxed when the back muscles are in spasm. A final warning: for people with very painful headaches and very thick hair, without first shaving the area, it is impossible to adhere the sensor directly on painful areas with any chance of getting good readings. Needless to say sensors are never placed on the area of the head covered by hair.

Awareness

Biofeedback is a very useful tool because the sensors do let us see and help understand how our body reflects its comfort and discomfort. When the body aches, it is dif-

ficult to know how tense we are and it is then that biofeedback becomes useful. It is also encouraging to monitor
our progress from visit to visit. When the system indicates
tension, it helps us understand tension is one reason for
the pain. It confirms that our pain is real. This can be very
reassuring for those of us being told our pain is "only psychosomatic" and created in our "head"! Biofeedback contributes to awareness. Awareness is the first step towards
managing stress and, visit after visit, biofeedback shows
progress made in controlling stress. Biofeedback becomes
an ally by showing us that we are on the right track.

HYPNOSIS to become free

Hypnosis, from a Greek word meaning sleep, can be useful in reducing tension and pain. There is nothing terribly
scary about hypnosis which, sectarian myths aside, is nothing more than a guided meditation that holds a suggestion
and invites you to improve. Have you ever seen children
watching television and ignoring the rest of the world? Or
playing video games and totally ignoring someone calling
them? People with chronic pain can go into a "trance" just
as these children do, and can become hypnotized simply
by practicing deep breathing and visualization. Hypnosis
is a state of altered consciousness that occurs normally just
before we enter into the sleep state.

Short history of hypnosis

Hypnosis is not new. Numerous ancient religious practices brought altered states of consciousness. These approaches date back to the ancient Egyptian and Hebrew healers
and to the Assyrio-Babylonian physician-priests using
magical rites, chanting, breathing exercises and meditations several thousand years before Christ. These same
practices are found also in Buddhist, Hindu, Shinto, Sufi

and early Christian meditations. Ancient Greeks had similar methods. Hippocrates and Plato confirmed its effects, along with Greek and Roman healing temples dedicated to Aesculapius, the god responsible for healing. These buildings contained a therapy room where priests would induce a state of deep relaxation and hypnosis through imagery and suggestions to cure the ill.[47]

Franz Mesmer was the first westerner to use hypnosis for healing and the word *mesmerism* for treatment by hypnosis comes from his name. Benjamin Franklin investigated Mesmer's approach and rejected it as "all in the patient's head". In 1784 a commission, set up by the Académie des Sciences, investigated Mesmer's work again and concluded imagination is effective and should be used. Only recently this recommendation was considered in the western world. Sigmund Freud, the neurologist who became the father of modern psychotherapy, supported hypnosis and used dreams if patients were unable to be hypnotized. In 1955 the British Medical Association approved hypnosis as a recognized form of treatment.[48]

However modern physicians (who are often scientists) and many clients prefer to use medications which are less expensive and appear to provide quick results. This is unfortunate because using only medication therapy does not produce the kind of personal growth often realized by hypnosis. The ideal course of treatment is to combine needed medication and hypnosis to produce permanent results.

A controversial therapy

Why do some people have doubts about hypnosis? Hypnosis is a controversial clinical treatment, mainly because it remains poorly researched. For centuries it has been identified as spiritualism, superstition and various kinds of witchcraft. This idea has been strengthened because many who support its use "believe" in it with a near-religious fervor. Exaggerated claims made by undisciplined persons have lead to additional controversy. In addition, some doctors and psychiatrists doubt its value because Freud gave it up sixty years ago, and because they have had little or no experience with hypnosis in its modern form.

The hypnotic state is no more dangerous or strange than is the sleep state. Practitioners of stage hypnosis exploit the trance state and human suggestibility for entertainment purposes further biasing the public view of hypnosis. Here we are discussing the type of hypnosis practiced by ethical and qualified practitioners. No extraordinary dangers with this type of therapeutic hypnosis have been demonstrated to exist.

The hypnotic experience is so familiar and because clients may expect something startlingly different from hypnosis, they may feel discouraged when a trance is induced. Clients should remember that during hypnosis one is not anaesthetized, no one becomes unconscious, no one ought to be asleep. One's mind is active, thoughts are under one's own control and stimuli are perceived as usual. If not alone, one is in complete communication with the therapist. The common experiences reported are feelings of heaviness in the arms, and tingling in the hands and fingers. If you are habitually a deep sleeper, you may doze momentarily. If you are a light sleeper, you may feel completely awake. Usually, under hypnosis, I feel mildly relaxed and tend to be slightly passive. For a few minutes I don't worry about time or achievement. Afterwards I feel very peaceful and calm, and stressors that often add pain do not seem to affect me any more. Problem solving is easier and pain decreases.

Suggestions to decrease pain

During an altered or hypnotic state, we may focus our concentration on something pleasant. Our ability to accept suggestions, often presented as images connected to senses, is increased and we feel relaxed. Pain usually decreases and can even totally disappear with the appropriate encouragement. A form of guided hypnosis involves suggestions from yourself or your therapist leading you to decrease your pain (ie. having you focus on a favorite memory or turning a button to control your pain level). Some people easily become hypnotized by breathing deeply and listening to someone tell them that they are becoming more and more relaxed.

It is important to repeat no one is ever under the hypnotist's control during a trance or hypnotic state. A hypnotist cannot force you to do anything against your will while hypnotized. Suggestions are based on your imagination and not on the hypnotist's imagination; and above all, you are always conscious and aware.[50] In my own experience I may decide not to pay attention to the environment while in a trance.

During my hypnotic sessions, I am always awake and in control of what I do. At any time I may decide to stop it and leave. Counting, for me, is not necessary to get up and start to move in the chair. I select images important to me. Nothing is imposed by the hypnotist. I am free.

Do your share of work!

Hypnosis feels like listening to a story, daydreaming, being in a cocoon or being a child tucked into bed. The perception of pain decreases because tension decreases and the mind focuses on something other than suffering. Meditation, visualization and hypnosis are different relaxation techniques but they can be combined into the same relaxation exercise. Anyone whose mind works reasonably well and who is willing to develop self-care, take charge of recovery from pain, develop imagination, implement solutions to medical issues and make a commitment to learn these techniques can successfully follow any of these approaches.

The return of memories

During a hypnosis session, old memories may come back to you and you may experience many events from your past. Images may enter your mind spontaneously. This is normal and is said to be the unconscious material returning to you. Sometimes these old events can impact your pain by momentarily increasing it. For example, past emotional abuses may return to memory and this added emotional pain may add to physical pain coming from other sources. The answer is first to give the pain expression previously denied, and then to imagine these abuses and associated sadness going away through imagery. You are then free to concentrate on controlling your physical pain and, because depression and pain are linked together, mastering positivism will help decrease pain.

Most of the time hypnosis feels like being very relaxed, slightly numb and almost ready to sleep. To get benefits from hypnosis, you need to trust the therapist and to be open to suggestions that lead you to a feeling of wellness. It is also important to openly express your reactions both to treatment and to your therapist, no matter how unfounded, unfair and/or ridiculous these may seem. If, for any reason, you believe you should interrupt therapy, mention your desire to do so. Important clues may be derived from your reactions, dreams and resistances that will provide a deeper understanding of your inner issues. These issues, of course, should be addressed if you wish to become well.

If your therapist is a trained psychologist, you may be able to obtain a refund from a third party health insurance provider. After a few sessions with a professional, you should be able to practice hypnosis by yourself, possibly with the assistance of an audiotape. This is called self-hypnosis or auto-hypnosis. Hypnotherapists typically provide such tapes as homework. In a sense, all hypnosis is self-hypnosis.

Success from hypnosis, like from other forms of psychological relaxation, will depend on your willingness to be responsible for your recovery and health. If you prefer to hand over control of your pain therapy to your physician, your family or society, you may have little affinity for use of relaxation techniques to manage pain.[51] However, please, try to regain control and consider practicing relaxation techniques in order to keep your medication doses to a minimum.

Relaxation is easily made part of your daily routine. You can't fail and even if you don't benefit as much as you would like, your attempts are never lost. Hypnotherapy on children can be also very successful as children typically have a powerful imagination, love stories and believe them. In addition, competent hypnotherapy has no ill side effects.[52]

Self-hypnosis

Hypnosis can be practiced just like meditation and visualization. The three approaches are also easy to combine. If you wish to practice self hypnosis or auto-suggestion to reduce pain, first find a quiet and comfortable place where you will not be disturbed. Wear comfortable clothes. Soothing music can help you to relax faster. You may begin deep breathing to allow energy into your body and release toxins. When you feel you are ready, try concentrate on your goal (such as decreasing pain or relaxing). Closing your eyes may make it easier to concentrate. It helps to imagine being in a beautiful and warm place, removed from stressors. It helps also to see and feel what you are trying to obtain, such as happiness, peace and decreased pain. The body will become relaxed and you will feel more in control because energy follows intent. It also helps to imagine sensations of numbness, wellness and lack of pain.

When you want to leave the hypnotic state, you count slowly from ten (or five) to zero; visualize that you are becoming more and more alert and finally you open your eyes. Once you are aware of the feeling of reduced pain, it will be much easier, even outside a "normal wakened consciousness trance", to get this state of peace and decreased pain. A therapist may coach you a few times until you are able to practice self-hypnosis. As with other psychotherapeutic approaches, the key to hypnosis is practice, practice and again practice.

It is possible to combine hypnosis with imagery, however both techniques are independent. Hypnosis is "the induction of a particular state of mind, while imagery is an activity."[53] Imagery is one way to provide suggestions while in a hypnotic trance. These suggestions can be visual, auditory, tactile, or connected to smell. Activity peaks in areas of the brain different than with hypnosis, as hypnosis is a mental function. Imagery directly affects physiology and has great emotional power. Research into medical uses of imagery is still in its infancy.

The "inner self" in your sacred space

We have seen that meditation, including other techniques as visualization and hypnosis, brings calm, relaxation and has a physical impact on the body. Less known is that meditation allows awareness (also called mindfulness or enlightenment), and makes possible contact with the "inner self". The idea is that pain, lack of time and social conventions easily cause us to hide our authentic personality. This authentic personality may be revealed by meditation, making us aware of truth and allowing new ideas to present themselves in a calm and comfortable environment. Meditation also assists in developing mental and physical energies, bringing about a better understanding of ourselves as well as healing and access to an extraordinary or sacred space.

How to explain healing from meditation? Western physicians believe healing power comes from a shift in the function of the endocrine system. Eastern healers explain that healing comes from improved circulation of *chi* within the body, and others believe that both explanations hold some truth.[54] Meditation, visualization and hypnosis are, as we will see later on, ways to get in touch with a superior or divine force. The best evidence of this spiritual expansion is the fact that pain affects the body, the mind and the spirit. Meditation helps to rise above the pain, and above ordinary life.

YOGA and TAI CHI to improve energy flow

If you do not feel a great affinity for these mental therapies, you may want to try other physical relaxation techniques that combine breathing, focus, meditation and physical movement. Yoga is a Sanskrit word meaning "union of body, mind and spirit." This therapy brings the body and the mind together. It can be performed alone or in a group, and is becoming increasingly popular in western culture. Yoga requires positive thinking and allows one to transform fears or worries into positive thoughts.

Many benefits

The exercises of yoga are designed to put pressure on the glandular systems of the body in order to increase total health. This removes toxins from the body, cleanses the lungs, takes away compression in nerve pathways, and improves blood circulation and the flow of vital energy within and between the *chakras*. Breathing is considered to be the source of life and is important to health. Most yogic breathing exercises require slow, deep and long breaths inhaled through the nose and involve lifting up the chest and the diaphragm. Yoga exercises and breathing prepare the body and the mind for meditation. Over one hundred schools of yoga are known, each insisting on different techniques to obtain the same results. Hatha yoga is commonly practiced in Northern America.[55]

Yoga is based on the philosophy that vital energy is supplied from within the individual, whereas tai chi involves flowing movements combining positions essential for balance and flexibility. This balance includes both the emotions and the mind. Tai chi is designed to be a non-stressful use of physical movements, facilitating organ health, rather than emphasizing muscle strength. For this reason tai chi is considered to be an internal healing art. Its movement strengthens the immune system by increasing circulation throughout the body. Tai chi also places great emphasis in the mind/body relationship and aims at improved mental and physical health.[56] Both activities, yoga and tai chi, reduce pain and increase movement ability. They require the will to take responsibility for our healing, the commitment to practice on a regular basis, preferably daily, and they force you to decide to let go of worries and bad habits.

Our society teaches us that stressful habits are good if they result in success and money. Modern technology makes work even faster paced with immediate answers being requested by everyone. Competition is everywhere. This puts constant and strenuous demands on the nervous system. Even children, in addition to attending school, follow numerous extracurricular activities and are often involved with competitive sports. This type of lifestyle at all ages can exacerbate pain. If the healthy barely manages to survive, the ill and/or injured certainly can't cope with stressful physical, mental and emotional demands. Yoga and tai chi assist in lessening anxiety and regaining harmony that is lost in our lives.

The ancient therapy of yoga

Yoga began in India several thousand years ago, before written history. Stone carvings showing yoga positions dating back at least 5,000 years ago have been found in the Indus Valley. Yoga is older than Hinduism which incorporates a variety of yoga practices. It likely arrived in the United States in the late 1800s but only became popular in the 1960s as part of a popular trend toward embracing holistic practices originating in the East. Part of yoga's current popularity is also explained by the fact that yoga is not expensive to practice. Beginners learning yoga can take a class with an instructor, read or watch a video. Yoga requires only a quiet and warm room, a mat or carpet, loose clothing and a few cushions. While it is relatively easy to learn, however, yoga takes commitment. It is a combination of postures and exercises allowing well-being. In the same way as meditation and hypnosis, it "has the ability to bring about an altered state of consciousness". When we reach this state, the muscles relax, creating some distance between the participant and the pain.[57] Yoga is not just about stretching, as is commonly believed. It includes a physical component with postures and movements developing flexibility and improving circulation. It has mental and spiritual components which increase energy and reduce stress. Both components are essential to healing, and yoga by balancing the *chakras*, helps us to balance our life.

The fluidity of tai chi

Tai chi is a gentle Chinese martial art, with dance like movements, reducing stress and tension by properly directing the energy flow. I find relaxation very effective and achievable with tai chi, in part because I listen to repetitive accompanying Tibetan music. Tai chi demands that I concentrate on movements and position of the body in order to properly reproduce them. The tai chi movements are joint oriented since the joints are said to control the amount of energy moving through the body. Tai chi seems almost magical. It is a sort of fluid, balanced and complicate ongoing dance which does not involve the still positions found in yoga, and which requires and develops intense concentration and excellent memory. It is also a combination of calm and excited movements connected to invisible balls or threads.

The use of a mirror with tai chi is helpful to create a distance between our minds and our bodies as we watch in the mirror. The body is the vessel holding pain; watching it in the mirror allows a disassociation between our minds and the pain. Of course this is far from easy: Tai chi, like yoga, requires a long term commitment both to develop the necessary memory skills (to remember positions) and to continue the ongoing training necessary to maintain the required body positions. Tai chi promotes growth, cultivates energy and "helps you to strip away the armoring and open closed places allowing who you are to emerge, free from the limitations which keep you hidden, and vulnerable."[58] It is "a meditation in movement" with several hundred official moving positions.[59]

Tai chi is an exercise with movements of the head, eyes, arms, hands, body, and legs all done in coordination with the mind while breathing appropriately. The secrets of tai chi practice include tranquillity of the mind, while the body remains relaxed and agile. The results appear peaceful and graceful. Another secret is to gather the *chi* (energy or breath in Chinese) to penetrate the entire body, unify the strength of the whole body and develop the *chi* into spirit.[60]

Traditional Chinese medicine is based on the belief that the cosmos can be divided into the following Five Elements: fire, earth, metal, water and wood. The wood element controls the joints which are essential in tai chi. When the joints become stronger and work well, blood circulation improves.[61] Tai chi teaches fluidity of movement in order to accomplish little things in a gentle way so that the joints are protected. It encourages good posture and the ability to re-establish connection with the earth. Its approach is non-intellectual and deals with stress in a body-oriented way. People are not required to reveal their worries; they are asked to pay attention and explore their levels of comfort or lack of it. Stress is viewed as a sign of energetic imbalance. Therefore one of the goals of tai chi is to influence mental/emotional changes through the experience of moving the body. Stress is a mental/emotional situation expressed through the physical body. The breathing process affects the stress levels of the mind and emotions. However tai chi never intends to prescribe change or to promote particular body or mental state. Each individual is unique and their comfort levels are also unique.[62]

The origins of tai chi dates back to about 2,000 years before Christ. In the 13th century A.D. a Taoist monk named Chang Sang Feng developed what we now call tai chi. This martial art is divided in different styles and the Yang style is most common in North America. It has three different forms: the simplified form, the short form and the long form. According to the tai chi philosophy, a force called *chi* flows throughout the body and becomes blocked. In curing disease tai chi and acupuncture work by freeing up blocked energy. A *yin yang* image is used as the tai chi symbol. Healing comes from harmony within the body and this harmony is reflected in the dance movements of tai chi.[63]

DISTRACTIONS to enjoy life

How do Ben-Gay and Tiger Balm work? They provide a distraction of the mind by gently irritating nerves beneath the skin and stimulating the sensation of heat to calm an injured muscle. Which type of distraction will you select? What do you like to do? Gardening, playing music, singing, reading, writing, drawing, painting, knitting, watching movies, spending time with children...? Distractions can provide powerful ways to reduce pain. Some of them come fairly easily if you spend time with people and have many interests in life. Others are appropriate to a specific group of people (for instance, children in pain love to be told stories) or to a time of day (for example, reading a good book in bed to help fall asleep and prevent pain from occurring at night). Another distraction is visualizing from perspective outside the body and looking inwards towards any painful parts of the body. This creates a distance between us and the pain. In this way, we become a sort of stranger indirectly involved with our pain. The distractions which work the best for me are ones that combine the different senses, such as gardening. This activity touches all of the senses with the beauty and scent of flowers, the taste of herbs and vegetables, the sun or the rain, the wind on the face, the dew on the feet or the fingers, the wind chimes, or the birds. Gardening is magical. At night in bed or in the middle of January in Edmonton, I have my interior garden which is my summer garden preserved in secret in my mind and very easy to recall. I can reach it any time anywhere by only focusing on it. Also, time spent with children and people remains one of my preferred distractions because these activities touch the heart. The most wonderful one is to be able to recreate positive feelings and bring memories alive again when loved ones are absent. Do you know a song saying that real love comes after love? Good memories are excellent mental distractions that take you away from pain.

SPIRITUALITY to connect with the universe

Spirituality brings inner peace, harmony and a feeling of connectedness with the universe. These important key elements are required in a chronic pain management plan aiming at making peace with pain. Prayers based on a connection with a higher force and with other people with the same belief system are more effective than prayers practised only for beneficial results. People who are highly spiritual, are known to suffer less in response to pain.

Tension and loneliness feed the cycle of pain, reduce the pain threshold and increase suffering. However the concept of integrative medicine blends together meditation, breathwork and spirituality into one component keeping away tension and loneliness. Prayers have their place in this search for reducing pain but they should not entirely replace conventional medicine. The most effective texts followed in meditation are spiritual and include universal values. It is consequently difficult and useless to separate a mantra from a prayer.

Meditation allows universal and spiritual values to integrate the pain management plan. It helps "to achieve deep personal insights and to release much of the negative emotional energy" increasing pain.[64] Belief in a superior force protecting us is very reassuring and allows for a better recovery. Many people in pain will wonder why they are the ones to experience pain. This question is "one of the most fundamental of all spiritual questions about suffering, because spirituality is, essentially, the search for meaning."[65] If we find an answer to the question and a meaning for pain, suffering decreases and awareness develops. At the same time inner peace, connected to awareness of truth, replaces painful frustrations.

As you know, meditation is an excellent channel to find answers and reach awareness. Usually people with chronic pain who have reached a state of awareness, experience more moments when pain disappears or decreases. Pain tends to decrease when we find a positive meaning to pain. We do not take anything for granted. Ironically we seem to appreciate wellness more when it disappears or when we are at risk to lose it. Several agree that pain makes individuals more compassionate and oriented towards the needs of others. This connectedness also allows support and love to be received from others. Surely awareness makes the ones experiencing chronic pain different from others. Awareness resulting from pain and meditation allows a sort of new morality with rules and definitions of the good and bad based on experiences with fighting pain. This new morality does not come from medical theories and other conventional regulations.

Giving our help and hearts to others in pain, doing something good for others, not taking everything for granted, being a part of a larger universe, taking care of our health, enjoying pain free moments (the Latin *Carpe diem*), accepting the things impossible to change and pay-

> **Life is more accurately measured by the lives you touch than by the things you acquire.**
>
> Anonymous

ing more attention to spirituality, – all of these become priorities with the new morality born from pain. The link between spirituality and medicine is very ancient and has been proven in traditional cultures where the shaman, a spiritual authority, is also a medicine man. It is interesting to note that miracles are usually associated with recovery from illnesses or medical conditions. People who habitually pray, are more successful at decreasing their pain than other persons not trained to pray. Science is slowly acknowledging the link between prayer and healing.

What is happiness for the ones with chronic pain? Or what should it be? How do we know we are healed and can enjoy happiness? Healing and happiness are personal decisions. You can decide to get up in the morning and be happy, or you can decide to be miserable. Only you can decide for yourself. You recognize happiness in the little ordinary things becoming extraordinary in the space you have created around yourself to ensure your healing. It is up to you to decide that you want to be happy even in the most painful, darkest lonely moments.

Life in extraordinary space

Happiness is closing your eyes and listening to the birds at 3:00 am from your bed, enjoying their music when everyone in the house is asleep, and you are lonely, planting spring bulbs or summer lilies while you imagine the flowers you will nurture, looking with a friend for wild orchids in a river valley, repeating to yourself "there are no unsolvable problems, only challenges", and meditating on the idea that pain is only a perception, being able to imagine a park full of flowers you are going to enjoy before falling asleep.

Happiness is connecting well with a medical team supporting you forever in all situations, having the freedom to perform daily activities without assistance from other people, playing with children, walking under the rain to reduce inflammation of the nerves, looking at the sky and imagining the world from the clouds.

Happiness is being able not to think about next week or next month, not being scared by tomorrow, hugging children, having them walk slowly into your room in the middle of the night and joining you in bed, going for a walk each day and breathing fresh air, smelling the scent of apples, mint and mushrooms in the backyard, looking at the sun light playing on the fall leaves.

Happiness is thinking you are an important part of the universe even if you do not know the rest of the world, believing there is always someone who cares for you even if this person is invisible, remembering the most essential is invisible to the eyes and visible only to the heart.

Happiness is eating chocolate with children, visiting the local market and enjoying the smells of life, reading a book on flowers or listening to a symphony, taking a pink bubble bath, asking a friend to rub your back, holding something warm in your hands.

Happiness is having intimacy in an extraordinary space, trying to guess what people feel and do not say, looking for rainbows or counting small snowflakes on the window.

Happiness is about doing ordinary things, with people who care, in a space you decide that is extraordinary. Happiness is to live with rules and definitions of the good and the bad based on your own experiences with constant chronic pain. To be at peace with pain is to learn from the ordinary, to recognize, disclose and wash away with tears the buried painful issues poisoning us in the hidden parts of our lives. To be at peace with pain is also to accept pain and to develop a positive mission from it rather than to fight it. It means focusing on the present, feeling how pain feels at the moment and understanding that pain needs not preclude living now. Then it is easy to believe pain will not prevent living and enjoying future moments.

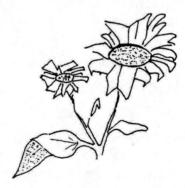

Chapter 5

ENERGY MEDICINE

Definitions

Energy medicine does not separate body from mind; it gives power to the ones with pain and is not invasive; it takes into consideration emotions and does not involve many scientific interventions; it often relies on the therapist's intuition. It connects us with past experiences and helps to solve inner issues impacting wellness. It is also called fringe medicine or eternity medicine or non local medicine because it is limited neither by space nor by time. Of course it can be painful because it supports the idea that physical work is needed to erase messages causing symptoms and to treat injured tissues. Chinese medicine is a form of energy medicine.

> Energy is life. It is the invisible force that animates the human body and permeates everything in the natural world, including animals, plants, trees and rocks, as well as the earth, sun, moon and stars.
>
> Airey, *Healing energies*, 2003, p. 6.

Alternative medicine has a culturally dependent definition. North Americans use the terms to mean any non scientific medicine such as energy medicine or Chinese medicine. However a treatment considered to be alternative in North America may not be defined as an alternative form in Asia or Africa. In the same way, our scientific and conventional medicine may be perceived as alternative in other countries. Even in Northern America, some people support the idea that a treatment is alternative when others consider it conventional because some Oriental therapies are quickly accepted by our scientific system. In a controversial field such as chronic pain, where different expert opinion is the norm, the best decision is to keep an open mind. Different treatments from various origins are worth consideration. It is for you to assess the results and select that which is the most appropriate for you.

ALTERNATIVE OR INTEGRATIVE OR COMPLEMENTARY?

Disagreement among experts notwithstanding, the domain of alternative medicine involves professionals who are experts in the treatments they offer. Any form of medicine can be dangerous. Any type of treatment may fail. Positive outcomes may prove elusive if expert opinion is missing. Experimenting with herbs without knowing the effects or correct doses for the specific condition being treated is one such risk. Acupuncture requires years of study and practice to achieve expertise, likewise with herbal therapy using plants. You would do well to check your therapist's qualifications and/or talk to other persons being treated by the same therapist to assess their qualifications and levels of expertise.

Unfortunately, alternative treatments have little quality control and may not be well reimbursed by third party insurance carriers. Finally cost may become burdensome for the one with pain. In spite of all this, many alternative treatments have been developed over hundreds of centuries by many thousands of people, and may well bring real relief.

Of course it is often useful to combine alternative treatments with conventional medical practises. You may decide to take pharmaceutical medication and practice meditation or be treated by an acupuncturist. The number of North Americans using alternative treatments is increasing while the number of family doctors – pillars of our medical systems – is unfortunately decreasing. At the same time increasingly improved pharmaceuticals are available from highly specialized physicians and these medications, even if not well tested over prolonged periods of time, have fewer nasty side effects. Maybe a good solution is to get the best treatments from both alternative and conventional medicines.

What you want is to decrease your pain, and using medications and other treatments that give you the best results (placebo or not) is always valid, regardless of the nature of medical theories and user feedback. Perhaps alternative or energy medicine holds the solutions for you and perhaps these can be combined with our conventional North American medicine. This approach is called "integrative" or "complementary" medicine and it is a current trend followed by the ones with pain who like ourselves, appreciate having a sense of control.

You should be aware that a debate is currently taking place in our western society. Several North Americans started to support traditional Chinese medicine as a reaction to a very medicated society asking science to solve medical problems and also selecting medications to treat unwelcome emotions, at the same time by reducing personal work as well as responsibility. These lifestyle medications, often changing emotions with unknown long term effects, treat depression, sadness, anxiety and other unwanted moods. They are heavily advertised and marketed among physicians prescribing them. In addition, few people, in our busy North American society, have time for personal development by mental therapies. This means some people support scientific medicine and others prefer energy medicine. If you select one rather than the other, you will feel pressure for your choice and most probably you will be criticized for your decision. So, please do not forget this is your life and you are entitled to make decisions you believe to be the best for you. You may also want to try both medicines according to your needs and circumstances. Energy medicine, as well as mental therapies, are usually more time consuming than scientific medicine using mainly medications.

BE IN CHARGE AND HEAL YOUR LIFE!

Therapists offering alternative medicine usually take longer periods of time to talk to you, during consultations, and to know you. Their aim is usually to care for you as a whole person and to concentrate only on the causes of the pain. In some respect they follow Hippocrates who wrote that it was more important to know the person needing medical care than to know the disease.[1] This attitude is usually very

> *Alternative medicine may not cure your pain – but it sure could heal your life.*
> Dillard, 2002, p. 2.

attractive to the ones with chronic pain because pain affects all aspects of the ones experiencing it in addition to affecting the lives of those living around the ones with pain. Therapists practising alternative medicine will probably try to bring harmony, balance and peace to you if you agree to be actively in charge of your health and recovery.

ORIENTAL MEDICINE

We include under the name of alternative medicine treatments developed to change or improve the energy force within the person needing care. Energy force flows through every living thing, including the human body. It is called *prana* in India and *chi* in China. In the west it is called orgone or bioenergy. It is invisible however essential to health. The electromagnetic energy field of the earth impacts our body and when our individual energy does not move freely as it should, we suffer from pain and become ill. Pain is linked to unbalanced energy and appears at certain points in the body as a way to catch our attention and communicate something is wrong. Recovery is reached when energy becomes free through therapies including physical and mental exercises, acupuncture, light, colour, plants or crystals.

Numerous and complex Chinese and Indian traditions are based on the energy concept at the centre of Oriental medicine. If this life force is balanced, the body is healed and functions well. Chinese practices also classify food by energetic values rather than by calories or fat component. Energy medicine indicates which areas are unbalanced and treats areas where the pain is located. It does not treat the actual pain but rebalances energy and works in harmony with the body natural healing ability.

Chi is similar to the immune system in western medicine. It nourishes and defends the body against disease, and runs through the body along energy channels (often called meridians) which are similar to arteries and veins. There are a total of 12 main meridians in our body including six *yin* and six *yang*. There are about 365 acupuncture points along the meridians where *chi* is concentrated.[2] When it is obstructed, *chi* can be manipulated by acupuncture, massage, meditation or self-hypnosis.

Yin and yang

An essential component of Chinese beliefs is the *yin* and *yang* which are opposing but complementary energies producing the life force or *chi*. The *yin* and *yang* must be balanced to restore or maintain health and to allow *chi* to flow normally. According to Taoist philosophy, our two energies, *yin* and *yang*, are different but interdependent. They represent our emotions and challenges. Each has a different meaning and is connected to the five elements -fire, wood, earth, water and metal – that are at the base of the universe.

Yin	Yang
Bottom part of the body; right side of the body; right part of the brain	Upper part of the body; left side of the body; left part of the brain
Emotions, feelings, interior life	Force, authority, exterior life
Moon, winter, water, cold, night	Sun, summer, fire, hot, day

Woman, family, society, business that protects and allows a living, dark, black	Man, individualism, hierarchy, authority, clear, white
Lungs, heart, kidney, liver	Stomach, intestine, bladder

Source: Odoul, 2002, p. 78 – 129.

Health results from a balance between *yin* and *yang*. Each part of the body derives its meaning from its connection to *yin* or *yang*. Pain is a symbolic sign or message coming from our unconscious and has a meaning for us to discover. Symbols attached to *yin* and *yang* assist in getting a better understanding of this meaning. It is important to understand the meaning of our pain if we want to make changes that allow us to heal.

A Chinese physician interviews you extensively; he or she asks questions on your pain, your physical symptoms, your food, your sleep, your emotions, your family and your life in general. The physician observes, listens and smells during the examination in order to assess your health. Your pulse is taken a few times because the physician gets from this examination various details on your internal organs and your health. He or she takes six pulses in each wrist on specific points on arteries corresponding to organs such as the heart, liver and kidney. Pulse taking is one of the most important diagnostic tools in Chinese medicine. It requires several years of training and practice. A Chinese physician also studies your tongue, its color, shape, size, coating and texture, in order to get additional information on your medical condition. Each part of the tongue corresponds to an organ. The therapist will then suggest different treatments: acupuncture, deep tissue massages, moxibustion (application of small mounds of burning herbs), cupping (suction cups). A combination of these treatments may be prescribed. A Chinese physician often also prescribes a strong tea or extract or pills made from various herbs and ingredients that will remain unknown to you. He or she may suggest martial arts or exercises, such as tai chi, combining breathing, movements and some meditation. All these treatments unblock the flow of energy and treat organs. Clinical diagnosis and treatment used by Chinese physicians are based on taking care of symptoms and syndromes. This medicine is unique and totally different from western medicine. However it has been used for several thousands of years and it is one of the official medical sciences of the world.

THE MEANING OF OUR PAIN

What does the body want to tell us? Opinions vary, and we want to lay down no hard and fast rules. However humans have 7 cervical vertebrae and this number is considered to be spiritual. There are 7 *chakras*, 7 planets, 7 colors in rainbows and 7 musical notes. The 7 cervical vertebrae hold what is the most essential in our body which is our head (with the brain controlling the body).[4] Bones represent our structure and relationship with life. Pain in the vertebrae and bones indicates pain in our internal structures and deepest beliefs. The specific point where pain originates also has a meaning. Pain in the legs means tense relationships with people or someone because legs allow motion and contact with others. Hips support and control our legs. They allow motion and flexibility. Pain in the hips implies lack of internal support; pain in the left hip indicates loss of a male figure (husband or father, *yang* symbol) and in the right hip, loss of a female figure (wife or mother or family, *yin* symbol). The knees are joints that are easy to bend and represent acceptance or obedience. Pain in the knees indicates refusal to accept an emotion or an idea. The side, left or right, would explain if this issue is caused by a relationship with a *yang* or a *yin* element.

The upper part of the body indicates action and consequently power (*yang* symbol). Pain in the arms means tensions in our desire to do or select something. Pain in the shoulders that control the arms, suggests difficulties in a desire to do when the exterior world does not give us means to achieve something. The side, left or right, *yang* or *yin*, gives clues to have a better understanding of the difficulties. Pain in the nape of the neck indicates difficulties or the impossibility to make real ideas or wishes. A stiff neck appears when we are unable to say no or refuse things.

Our organs have also interpretive meanings. Pain in our stomach suggests worries, liver problems are connected to anger, and kidney issues refer to our fears. Our heart, closely connected to our brain, is the home of love and emotions. Physical issues found in the heart remind us of our difficulties with love and emotional management. Our brain is the body's central computer. Physical problems relating to the nervous system indicate our difficulties as we use thoughts while managing our life. These issues are also an indicator that we find it difficult to make space for joy. They are a sign of our difficulty in transferring our thoughts and desires into something real.[5]

CHAKRAS:
REAL EVEN IF OUTSIDE WESTERN MEDICINE

Energy enters through and flows inside the spine through the *chakras* which correspond to points along the spine. They control our physical health, emotions and attitudes. This belief was born in India, and has been followed for thousands of years. Each *chakra* controls internal organs and systems. The word *chakra* means wheel in Sanskrit and each acts in synchronicity with the endocrine system. Each one controls and nourishes a part of body and has specific characteristics.

Three *chakras* are found in the abdomen, at the base of the spine, just below the navel and the ribcage, connected to the energy of life (survival, sexual and social interaction and self-confidence). The legs and feet are extensions of the abdominal *chakras*. The thoracic cavity protects the heart and lungs, and houses two *chakras* attached to relationships and love, one being the heart *chakra* for unconditional love and the other being the throat *chakra* for communications. The heart *chakra* is attached to the arms and hands for reaching out and hugging, and the throat *chakra* is responsible for the ears and mouth (communicating). Two *chakras* are housed in the head, one between the eyes and one above the head, and are related to the energies of awareness, wisdom and light.[6] The *chakra* located between the eyes is attached to the top vertebra in the neck by a muscle extending across the head from the top of the neck to the forehead. In my own experience, massaging the top of the neck helps to reduce pain between the eyes. You look after your own *charkas* with deep breathing, proper nutrition and exercises, massages of their locations and meditation.

Chakras are associated with particular colors, and have

a vibrational frequency. Being ill indicates that the energy levels are blocked or drained and should be raised and opened. Many factors can cause energy blockage and damage *chakra* balance. These include stress, physical and mental pain, lack of sleep, of rest and exercise, poor diet, pollution, allergies, negative environment with little love and support, unrealistic demands at home and at work, and changes in personal lifestyle. These conditions have an impact on both the quality and quantity of the energy we absorb and give out. No one can prevent these stressors completely and each of us should pay attention to them.

Chronic pain is complex, uses a very high volume of energy and causes a lack of balance. This makes it necessary to release blocks in the *chakras* and subtle bodies through appropriate treatment. A pendulum can be useful to check which *chakras* are out of balance or to confirm that all are open after treatment. Several therapies used in energy medicine will be suggested to rebalance energy and calm the mind and body in order to improve resistance and achieve peace with pain. Pain reduction is a consequence of rebalancing energy and is not the main goal of medical intervention.

Here is a table illustrating the nature and role of the seven *chakras*:

Chakra	Colour and sound	Controls	Connected to
First or Root, base of the spine	Red (mantra, called also healing sound: "lam")	Ovaries, skeletal structure, large intestine and lower body	Physical survival, security, ambition, financial situation

Second or Sacral, just below the navel	Orange (mantra: "vam")	Reproductive system, bladder and circulation	Sexuality, creativity, feelings, emotions, pleasure
Third or Solar plexus, just below the ribcage	Yellow (mantra: "ram")	Adrenal glands, spleen, pancreas, stomach	Identity, self-confidence, courage, power, ability to make right decisions
Fourth or Heart, centre of the chest	Green (mantra: "yam")	Thymus gland, immune system, glands	Compassion, unconditional love, relationships
Fifth or Throat	Blue or turquoise (mantra: "ham")	Thyroid gland, lymphatic, immune and neurological systems	Trust, self-expression, communication, learning
Sixth or Third eye, centre of the brow on forehead	Indigo (mantra: "om")	Pituitary gland, central nervous system	Intuition, understanding, perception, clarity and insight, spiritual knowing, psychic abilities
Seventh or Crown, at or just above the top of the head	Violet (mantra: none, silence) or gold or transparent as a clear crystal	Pineal gland	Higher energies and spiritual realms, openness, maintains overall balance of the *chakra* system, channels universal energy into the body

Table adapted from Airey, *Healing Hands*, 2003, p. 35 and *Healing Energies*, 2003, p. 43.

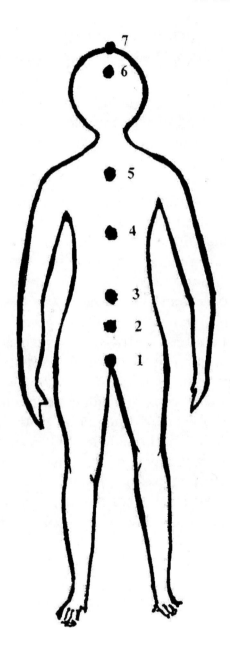

The Seven Chakras

Why take care of the chakras?

Various texts provide detailed information about *chakras* and it is beyond the scope of this book to provide an exhaustive account. The first *chakra* is red and entails all issues attached to practical skills, survival, reality of the present and immediate needs. Problems with physical movement, such as strained ligaments, pulled muscles, misalignment, issues with colon, fatigue, and exhaustion are improved by balancing this *chakra*. The second *chakra* is orange and affects all types of flow within the body, that of feelings and information, feeding cells, release of toxins and reproductive flow. Joint stiffness as well as infertility, constipation, water retention and indifference or lack of creativity come from blocked energy in this *chakra*. The third *chakra* is yellow and houses the power station in the body. It contains the digestive system and major nerve centres. Stress, anxiety, intolerance to foods and chemicals, loss of enthusiasm, inability to focus, and bad memory are indications that this *chakra* requires attention. The fourth *chakra* is green (which is the middle of the spectrum of light). It is found in the middle of the body and in the centre of the *chakra* system. It is then not surprising to find there lie the balance, harmony and equilibrium at all levels. When we suffer from anxiety, lack of hope and a feeling of being trapped, we should balance the energy in this *chakra*. The fifth one is blue and controls throat issues, tightness in the neck and shoulders, difficulties in communicating, making social adjustments, and being heard. The sixth *chakra* is violet or amethyst in color. It is called the third eye because it looks inside to understand while the two physical eyes look outwards. This third eye is very important and connects with imagination, creativity and dreaming. It finds hidden components visible only to this *chakra*. The third eye is "a psychic place at the threshold of the inner and outer worlds, and is a natural seat of knowledge."[7] This site between the eyebrows is linked to headaches, migraines, depression and stress, and issues with concentration and memory. The crown *chakra* is amethyst or clear without color. It allows energy to enter the body and controls the life force. It is also the centre for imagination, inspiration and unconditional service to the ones in need. Attention should be given to this site when one deals with conditions attached to loneliness, stress and lack of empathy. Care to the last *chakra*, connecting us to the entire universe, is also extremely important. Accounts with respect to color vary only at the top of the system, where the light spectrum passes out of the visible range.

Chronic pain is a considerably complex condition which can be affected at the physical, emotional and emotional levels by all seven *chakras* causing the symptoms attached to chronic pain. Consequently therapy will be required on the entire spine in order to be at peace with pain.

Oriental practices

Chinese physicians use different diagnostic practices than do western physicians. The tongue is an important source of information to understand the physical condition of the body. Pulse reading and assessment of body odour are also key sources to assess health. When Chinese physicians have a good understanding of their clients' physical conditions, they work on re-establishing harmony in their *chi* with treatments including acupuncture, massage and pressure sometimes applied with the use of their own body, such as elbows and knees. These medical practices are far from being gentle and they are generally painful, especially if the physicians decide to create an injury in order to force the body to heal through this injury.

It is probably fair to state that oriental therapies, including acupuncture, are techniques that may be approached with a western or an eastern mindset. western practitioners speak of endorphins and pain reduction. Eastern practitioners speak of energy, balance, release, and harmony.

Oriental therapies are very different from our North American medical traditions giving priority to decreasing pain at all costs while Chinese medicine aims at producing healing without necessarily killing pain. If you seek immediate pain reduction, you may not want to select Chinese medicine. Although we fully believe in our readers' ability to choose the nature of their treatments, we wish to warn there may be inconsistencies between selected therapies. You should also know that Chinese physicians may be unable to treat your injuries if you have been treated first by invasive western scientific medicine. This means that surgery impacting nerves, for example, may produce unwanted effects that might fall beyond the limits of Chinese medicine. Options should be assessed as early as possible for each condition; this is far from being easy when western medical practices, seeking to create a sense of well-being by severing the mind from the body, are at variance with Asian medical traditions.

SUBTLE BODIES: EVEN MORE CHALLENGING

The energy around the body can be seen as seven whirling wheels of colour or layers of light called "subtle bodies"; each of them has a specific function. Healing requires the *chakras* and the subtle layers to be properly aligned. These bodies can be easily summarized:

Name of subtle bodies	Definition
Etheric body	Closest to the physical body, provides a blueprint for the physical body
Emotional body	The seat of the emotions
Mental body	Mental activity, thoughts, ideas, daily concerns
Astral body	Representation of the personality
Causal body	Seat of willpower and gateway to higher consciousness, fulfilment of personal destiny
Celestial soul body	Spiritual essence, also called "higher self"
Illuminated spiritual body	Highest level, where we become one with the Divine or source of love and healing

Table adapted from Airey, *Healing Energies*, 2003, p. 10 and Lilly, 2003, p. 11.

Energy vibrating in the *chakras* and the subtle bodies is often invisible to the naked eye but can be felt as tingling by rubbing one hand against the other. We may perceive it when we believe our personal space is being invaded by someone coming too close to us or when we sense a presence without actually looking at the person.

Oriental medicine is also based on the twelve meridians conducting energy to and from the cells and organs, bringing nourishment and removing toxins. They start and end in the hands and feet. Diseases appear when a meridian is blocked and different techniques using pressure or stretching can be applied to release blocked energy and reopen them.

PENDULUM, A MATTER OF FAITH

This is a healing tool made with a small object, attached to a thin chain, which provides a diagnosis or some information about physical or mental state. A crystal is often used in the making of a pendulum but any heavy material such as wood and metal may also be used. The movement of a pendulum, which is held with two fingers and slowly carried over the spine and head, can indicate the energy state of specific *chakras*. Different energy states in the client's *chakras* interact with the healer's aura, causing the pendulum to move in distinctive ways. If a *chakra* is blocked and does not work properly, the pendulum held above this *chakra* does not move and indicates the source of a health issue. This unhealthy condition should then be treated. Pendulums provide by their movement a positive or negative answer to a clear question connected to the health of the one needing care. The particular movement that indicates a "yes" or a "no" answer needs to be established by the practitioner through meditative practice with the pendulum. Questions can help to find the source of pain and when this is known, healing becomes possible. The same inquiries can be repeated to check the accuracy of the answers. Better results are obtained if the client lies on his or her back when the healer places the pendulum over the *chakras*.

The therapist does well to spend some time alone with the pendulum, before working with a client, in order to determine how the pendulum will move for positive and negative answers. This knowledge will assist the healer in interpreting any movements. The motion indicating a yes or a no is consistent for everyone. The healer must therefore ask the pendulum to indicate a positive and a negative response. The pendulum is activated by the client's energy and by the healer's intuition. Pendulum dowsing requires a very large dose of faith and openness to new therapies. Anyone can try it and obtain good results with a little practice. Even people living with pain can do this and achieve results provided that an open mind is maintained during the process.

HEART-CENTERED THERAPY, A NEW APPROACH TO CHRONIC PAIN

Heart-centered therapy is not a cure but rather a trusting connection and interaction between someone suffering from chronic pain and a therapist or healer providing care and unconditional love. This relationship includes non traditional techniques, such as hypnotic suggestion, deep breathing or visualization. The connection involves sharing the burden of pain and giving someone compassion, respect and unconditional love. The most important part of the therapy is to be oneself with the caregiver, without being judged or forced to pretend feelings of benefit to others, and to have a privileged healing relationship with the therapist. Solutions to address issues and reduce suffering are discussed and implemented by the client. Deep breathing, visualization and hypnosis are used as tools to extract unconscious sources of suffering and pursue possible solutions for implementation. The positive sharing of energy, at the base of this therapy, leads to healing and an improved quality of life. The ones with pain know they have support and someone reliable if needed. This is important because several physical and mental therapies, such as acupuncture, massages, physiotherapy, chiropractic care and visualization increase pain before reducing it.

This therapy should not come as a surprise because care and love are two different translations of the same concept. People suffering from chronic pain look for care rather than a cure, as is so well expressed in the words "health care." The therapists need to remove traditional barriers separating health care providers from their clients, and provide a good level of support of the ones in pain. The therapist giving and the client receiving therapy should be able to have affinities to build a partnership and develop a long term connection. The development of relationships may take time and is not always quickly achieved.

> **The client is the proprietor of the entire process.**
> Sussman, 2002, p. 116.

Those receiving therapy do a part of the work. They should be prepared to share previous painful physical and emotional experiences, and ultimately must trust the therapist if they agree to pursue psychotherapy. Sometimes it may be necessary to develop a healthy life style including new exercises, meditation, breathing exercises and other known pain reducing activities. Heart-Centered Therapy is not traditional but about 80% of the world's population uses non- traditional medicine with a very high degree of success.

ACUPUNCTURE, ANOTHER COMPLEX THERAPY

Acupuncture is one of the most ancient therapies and has been practiced in Asia for thousands of years. In China, this therapy is very conventional, however, in North America, it is considered to be an alternative therapy very often rejected by insurers. It was introduced to the west in the 17th century by a Dutch physician and was mentioned as a successful treatment in 1823 by a British medical journal. It became popular in North America and England in the early 1970's when contacts were developed with China.[8] In Taoist terms, acupuncture removes excess or deficient *yin* or *yang* energies and it gets rid of blocks in the energy flow.

The term includes the Latin word *acus* or needles that are the tools used in this therapy. Very fine needles are inserted into the skin to stimulate or reduce the energy force or *chi*. They remain in the skin for a few minutes, and several needles are usually used per session. The therapist may twist the needles, connect them to an electric current, or put a piece of burning incense on the end. This treatment is said to relax the entire body and can be an excellent method in reducing pain. Unfortunately, as with any alternative treatment, therapists do not all have the same training or offer the same quality of therapy. Acupuncture is more effective when the therapist has many years of experience and the client believes it will offer relief. Arthritis is a condition often treated by acupuncture with a good rate of success. In my specific case, acupuncture did not bring much benefit. This can be attributed to a number of reasons: injured muscles and other soft tissues stiffen at the time of contact, the muscles going into spasms and thus rejecting the needles. The muscles would become very hard and it would then take me several hours of heat and stretching to relax. Please note that many people achieve good success from acupuncture treatments.

People experiencing chronic pain should attempt acupuncture therapy more than once because of its high degree of success at treating pain. However according to western research, people suffering from pain caused by nerve damage, such as in cases of diabetes, alcoholism, toxic nerve injury, and kidney failures, usually do not experience relief with acupuncture.[9] Therefore acupuncture should be attempted however it may not be the best solution for any one case. In my own experience I found it very painful, even though I used pain reducing techniques, such as deep breathing or self hypnosis, during each acupuncture treatment.

Increased pain attached to acupuncture is normal because Chinese medicine aims at healing your body and your life; its primary goal is not to decrease pain. Chinese culture does not seem to consider reduced pain as a sign of wellness. Of course this does not mean Chinese medicine is not valid; we mean it is different from North American medicine. If your practitioner speaks like a western medical modeler, you might seek someone with a more eastern approach.

In western circles, it is believed acupuncture creates activity in the fast pain fibers that help to release endorphins, our natural painkillers. The treatment could also help the body to release steroids which may decrease pain.[10] Insurers have begun to cover acupuncture treatment, however most companies have a fixed maximum annual coverage. Chronic pain clients often end up paying for acupuncture as it usually requires repeated treatments quickly terminating benefits refunded by insurances. These insurance companies tend to welcome western practitioners almost exclusively.

FENG SHUI TO CLEAN UP YOUR SPACE

This Chinese practice, older than 1,000 years, involves environmental influences on health. *Chi* flows through the physical body, and also moves throughout the universe and along energy paths. Feng shui gives a harmonious environment where *chi* moves smoothly and where *yin* and *yang* are well balanced. Furniture with curves and soft drapes hold *yin* energy; straight drapes and bright colors spread *yang* energy. Harmony in the environment is essential to healing. Feng shui promotes the idea that we are healthier when we live in the same range of vibrations as the earth. Synthetic materials, microwave ovens and electrical equipment create negative energy while plants and crystals create positive energy. In my experience most people feel better in a room with flowers. Interior plants refresh the environment and add beauty to their surroundings. If your teens suffer from chronic fatigue and sleep in a cluttered room, their lack of energy may be partly caused by negative *chi* being released by a messy environment. Since most teenagers prefer to live in a clutter, one solution is to offer a plant for their room even though you may have to be the one to water it.[11]

MAGNETOTHERAPY, A MIRACLE CURE

Magnets, which have been used in healing since the ancient Greek and Chinese civilizations, can work to reduce pain and inflammation caused by a wide range of medical conditions, including injuries, arthritis and fibromyalgia. They are inexpensive, safe and often provide good results. Magnetic fields have an impact on the body's energy. Magnets are said to speed healing, facilitate the blood flow, reduce muscle spasms, improve oxygen supply to the cells, increase energy and stimulate the creation of nerve endings and the elimination of waste. They enhance the release of enkephalins which are chemicals similar to endorphins produced by the body and they reduce pain. No one really knows this is achieved even though many users, therapists and physicians believe they provide positive results.[12]

> Atoms, cells, human beings, the earth – all are charged with magnetic energy. So are the push and pull of weather patterns in the hemispheres, the movement of sun and stars.
>
> Lawrence, Rosch, Plowden, 1998, p. XVIII.

Increased circulation is an important result for the treatment of pain because it facilitates the removal of lactic acid from muscle tissues and decreases swelling caused by inflammation.[13] In some American statistical studies, magnets help between 80% to 99% of the users. They should not be used if the cause of pain is unknown because pain is a warning signal something is wrong in the body.[14] In our experience magnets can also be used as an adjunct to medication in order to maximize the effect of medications. Generally any increase in blood flow will decrease pain.

Magnets are used in mattresses, seat covers, shoe insoles, straps, wristbands and jewellery. They can be placed directly at the site of pain or on specific acupuncture points. If used on fractured bones, healing time may be shortened. Magnetic products provide good long term results if the strength of the magnet is therapeutically sufficient. Unfortunately the quality of magnets used in many products is not possible to verify prior to purchase.[15]

Therapeutic magnets are imprinted with north and south polarity labels, and a protective coating prevents breakage. The magnet's strength is essential and is measured "by a gauss meter in gauss units (oersted) or by the iron-weight it can lift, which is more approximate." For example, a two pound iron weight lift has a 500-600 gauss power. Large magnets are said to penetrate more deeply. The strength of a magnet depends on its size, weight and the materials used, while pain relief is dependant on the client's health, type of illness and power of the magnets.[16]

Ancient Chinese written records dated back to 2000 B.C. explain that magnetic stones placed on specific body parts cured imbalances and the Vedas – old religious texts from the Hindus going back to the same date – refer to "instruments of stone" treating disease. A Greek legend describes how Magnes, a shepherd living in Magnesia, discovered the power of these stones. The Greek philosopher Aristotle reported in writing on the therapeutic impact of magnets on the body and around 200 B.C., the Greek physician Galan recorded that pain could be reduced with magnets. Egyptian physicians also mentioned the therapeutic use of lodestones, and Romans treated arthritis and gout with the electric charge produced by eels. Two European physicians, Paracelsus (1493-1541) and Mesmer (1734 to 1815) believed magnets facilitated healing and had an impact on the life force. Many other scientists and healers, including Louis Pasteur, Pierre and Marie Curie, and Samuel Hahnemann who founded homeopathy, and the physicist Albert Einstein, studied and recommended the use of magnets in treatments.[17] Hahnemann "recognized magnetic energy as a principle of homeopathic effectiveness" since homeopathy most probably attracts "negative magnetic energy to the injury."[18] In spite of this extensive background, many persons experiencing pain do not view magnets as a possible beneficial therapy. Japan is the largest user of magnetic therapy, with about 30 million of magnets in use.[19]

Technology brings good news to those who are slow to trust alternative therapies. Kirlian photography and Vega testing monitor energy patterns and, in a sense, make them real to the human eyes. Kirlian photography provides an image of the energy pattern. If the energy level is high, the Kirlian picture is radiant with a smooth and even contour. If the person with chronic pain lacks energy, the Kirlian photograph may show no image at all or the photo may present an erratic outer edge or thin pattern. These tools reveal that illnesses, energy blocks, and physical and emotional conditions negatively impact on the energy level, while therapies help increase it.

Kirlian photography is a method measuring energy and viewing auras. It was discovered in 1939 by Semyon Kirlian, a Russian electrician, who found how to produce an image of the electromagnetic energy field surrounding the human body. He established contact between the human electromagnetic field and a high-voltage, high frequency electric charge. This provides an interference pattern which can be photographed. It is believed that image is produced if and where the body is out of balance. This method gives the best results with the body's energy taken near the hands and the feet.

Vega testing uses electronic devices which measure electrical properties on acupuncture points while the client grasps an electrode making a complete circuit. The Vega machine was developed in the 1970's by Dr. Helmut Schimmel. This equipment measures fluctuations in the body's magnetic field and indicates areas requiring therapy.[20] Although magnetic therapy is considered unconventional in North America, MRI (magnetic resonance imaging) scans are regularly used to investigate physical pain. This medically accepted technology is based on images of the body's magnetic energy.

REIKI, THE SCIENCE OF CARING HANDS

The word reiki means universal (*rei*) life force (*ki*) in Japanese. The term has its origins in Tibetan Buddhism. This form of therapy channels healing energy through the hands. It was rediscovered in Japan in the 19th century by Dr. Mikao Usui who repopularized it. Reiki is attached to sacred knowledge and to the tradition of master and student. However anyone willing to understand reiki can channel positive energy.

Reiki can be explained by first presenting the principle that the universe holds energy flowing through space and time, and also through anything on earth. People are connected to the universe and hold energy allowing life and well-being. Love is part of the energy. Through love and caring hands, this therapy rebalances the body's energy, and thus restores health.[21] People receiving reiki report that it is very relaxing, which is a sign of unblocked energy. Reiki therapists are said to feel the exchange of energy with their clients and to modify energy fields.[22] We should add that any time spent with a loving and caring person is always very useful in healing. If the mind feels good, physical healing often results from this well-being.

Reiki can be an excellent means to treat chronic pain connected with stress and physical injuries. Hands are applied on the *chakra* on the spine and the neck where the pain is located. I believe people in pain can use hands to gently press where it hurts. My own experience tells me this light pressure decreases pain. Since it can be painful to raise hands up on the neck or head, I like to practice reiki on myself while in bed, usually before falling asleep.

SOUND THERAPY TO SMOOTH YOUR LIFE

Sounds have a noteworthy impact on wellness. Music is well known to calm and bring about feelings of well-being while negative energies can be removed through healing sounds. It is also known that noise pollution causes stress.

Most people do not use their voice to decrease chronic pain unless they have been exposed to meditation. However chanting repeated mantra or words, and toning pure sounds with an unique and sharp note, as "a", "i," "u" repeated for a few seconds, clear the mind and bring healing energy. Singing (which can include chanting and toning) also decreases pain and fatigue. These activities release emotional trauma and promote good health. It is believed the subtle bodies, the *chakras* and the body vibrate at specific frequencies and if these vibrations become unbalanced, illness follows.

> *Sound therapy is one of the oldest and most profound forms of energy healing. From the simple repetition of mystical words to complex rhythms and structures, sound waves can alter our mood and enhance wellbeing.*
>
> Airey, *Healing Energies*, 2003, p. 46.

Sound therapy, with specific sounds at the same frequency as alpha and theta brainwave patterns, restores harmony.

Certain sounds with repeated rhythms, such as waves on a shore, or with high frequency, such as the ones produced by dolphins or birds, induce a state of well-being. Bells or gongs also produce healing sounds. High frequency sounds encourage the release of endorphins and can bring feelings of euphoria.[23]

Audiotapes with these sounds are recommended to remove tension, generate positive breathing and decrease pain. Tapes of nature sounds produce no side effects and are not expensive. They may remind us of holidays by the sea in exotic climates, or recall childhood memories.

> Close your eyes, start a journey through a strange, new world! Leave all thoughts of the world you knew before, close your eyes, let the music set you free...
>
> Andrew Webber, *The Phantom of the Opera.*

Music is essential at bed time when the mind can fill with thoughts or worries. Audiotapes can chase away negative energies, helping medications to achieve faster relief. They should become good companions at night to keep preciously at your bedside.

HOMEOPATHY, A SUCCESSFUL PARADOX TO SCIENTIFIC MEDICINE

Homeopathy, meaning "similar suffering" in Greek, encourages the body to heal by itself. Homeopathic preparations are made from plants, minerals and other natural products. The active agent is extremely diluted, and the energy of the active substance is said to remain in the "memory of the medicine." Homeopathic remedies with their high level of dilution are available without prescription. For example, allergy to bee stings is treated with formic acid (the toxin in bee stings). However, it is diluted to the point where the amount taken as medicine would not be expected to have even a single molecule of formic acid in it!

Homeopathy was developed in the 1700s by a German physician, Samuel Hahnemann, and is based on the premise that similarity cures similarity. In other terms, clients receive small doses of substances connected to the symptoms to be treated. For example, a skin rash can be treated with a very tiny amount of poison ivy. Homeopathic physicians believe that symptoms, such as fever, are not caused by the disease but by the body trying to heal. Consequently, a preparation providing fever will help the body to heal. Another component of homeopathy is to use small amounts of substances that support symptoms, such as a sedative herb to treat insomnia. The substances given to clients are meant "to stimulate the healing responses of their own bodies."[24] Ingredients are selected for matching a specific condition in an individual and are prepared by dilution and shaking leaving only a mere memory of the original components.[25]

Hahnemann began his experiments by consuming quinine used to treat malaria. He hypothesized that quinine caused him thirst, pain and fever, which are also symptoms of malaria. This experiment helped him to develop the "law of similars" and to publish *Organon of Rational Medicine* in 1810. He was criticized for his belief that homeopathic medicine was more effective if the dose of the treating ingredient was extremely small. This principle goes against scientific medicine where higher doses are said to produce better results.

Homeopathy is currently very popular in Europe. In England 42% of all physicians refer clients to homeopathic doctors, and according to the *British Medical Journal*, 81 of 107 reviewed trials showed positive results originating from homeopathy.[26] French medical schools offer courses in homeopathy and in this country where health insurance covers homeopathy treatments, one-third of all medical doctors employ a form of homeopathy in their practices.[27] Practitioners claim they can treat any diseases or symptoms, including chronic pain. There are now more than 3 000 homeopathic remedies made from plant, minerals and animal materials such as snake venom, squid ink and jellyfish. These ingredients are available in liquid, cream or pill form. Interestingly, we understand that the idea that water could hold a "memory" of something that once was dissolved in it, is consistent with recent advances in quantum physics. However, explanation of the healing benefits of homeopathy may be less esoteric than this. One of the reasons homeopathy works may be that physicians who use it, spend more time with clients, answering questions and preparing individualized medications.[28] This deeper relationship could explain the positive results from homeopathic treatments.

The connection between therapist and client is essential in homeopathy because practitioners believe that symptoms are specific to the client and not to the disease. This means two clients with the same set of symptoms can get different homeopathic preparations. In Canada and in the U.S. homeopathic medications can be found in health food stores. I would strongly recommend that you inform your physician about any homeopathic medication you plan to use because of possible side effects and interactions with your prescribed medications. Even if homeopathy is not widely used in North America, the World Health Organization gave it status of an approved traditional medicine. We believe this rich and diverse therapy can be effectively and efficiently combined with standard pre-scribed medications if you discuss your choice with your doctors.

NATUROPATHY, A FIELD TO EXPLORE

Naturopathy uses homeopathic preparations and naturo-paths employ various other treatments, including nutri-tion, massage, herbal medicine, exercise and hydrothera-py, to encourage natural healing and reduce suffering. This form of medicine was initiated by a German physician, Benedict Lust, who immigrated to the United States in 1892. Naturopaths treat the whole person, and may suggest modifications to the client's environment and promote a non-stressful lifestyle to prevent illnesses. They believe in a balanced, vital, natural force close to the Chinese *chi*. Naturopathic medicine, which is well-respected in Europe, can likely become more popular in North America in the upcoming years because of the increase in non-prescribed medications witnessed in this continent.

CRYSTAL THERAPY, THE CONTROVERSY

Crystals are believed to hold therapeutic qualities as they store energy from the earth, and are often recommend-ed by healers to decrease pain. They are very stable with a structure resistant to heat, pressure and other outside forces. Probably for this reason they are able to transform imbalances in our subtle energy system. Their meaning is taken according to their colours which reflect one of the seven *chakras*. Each colour holds a basic property.

Red crystals energize. They are attached to the bones and, since they are connected with the base *chakra*, they solve issues involving strained muscles or ligaments and misaligned bones. Amethyst and other cool colours, is said to be useful in meditation and to balance the energy bodies. It symbolizes the mind's control over the body and selfless service to others. Amethyst is the most powerful stone and has been used for centuries by crystal healers. It is said to be effective at soothing headaches. Symptoms should be noticed at an early stage in order to make them easier to heal. Indigo crystals that are matched with the brow *chakra*, can help heal headaches, migraines, depression. Indigo or dark blue crystals influence perception, understanding and intuition. Lapis lazuli and sapphire relax and bring peacefulness. They can be used for the brow and the throat *chakras*, the two sites where stress tends to accumulate. Rose quartz is believed to promote calm and release emotional blocks. Yellow gems relate to the solar plexus that contains major nervous centres, and preserve the body's nervous, digestive and immune systems. They are reported to remove stress. Amber has a positive impact on the nervous system and tiger's eye increases energy flow. Orange crystals, such as topaz and dark citrine, relating to the sacral *chakra*, are said to decrease joint stiffness. These gems are said to boost energy flow and treat blockages. Green stones are said to balance emotions and relationships, and encourage personal growth. Green, the colour of the heart *chakra*, love and hope, creates a feeling of relaxation and confidence. Blue crystals are attached to communications since blue is the throat colour. White stones and clear quartz are connected to the crown *chakra* and symbolize universality, clarity and purified energy.

Before using them in healing, crystals should be soaked

in a bowl of salt water over a period of a few hours to remove any negative vibrations. These gemstones are held by the therapist near the client or placed on the specific matching *chakras*. Earrings are another way to use crystals to cure painful and tense conditions in the neck, jaw and head. Stones can provide direct healing properties by physical contact or can be used in infusions, sometimes in association with a specific phase of the moon. This occurs when combined with "moon medicine" using the healing and calming energy of the moon. Crystal colours are an important part of moon medicine. Clear stones are associated with the full moon to enhance healing and darker or smoky stones with the waning moon to re-balance and clear negativity.[29]

What is true with crystal therapy? First of all, crystal therapy and moon medicine will work if you believe it will. This is called the placebo effect. Scientific studies indicate that in some clients, placebos can decrease pain. If you believe you are using healing therapy, you will begin to heal. The moon has a positive impact on mental and physical health. Scientific research is starting to investigate this effect.

We would be inclined to believe moon medicine may impact pain more than the crystals. Full moon is said to make people less rational and increases emotions. Even if you don't believe crystals can influence pain, gemstones are clear, colourful and magical in nature and will promote comfort, reduce tension and remind you to heal. Everyone needs a bit of magic to maintain hope in painful situations.

THERAPY WITH COLOURS TO MAKE YOUR WORLD BEAUTIFUL

Colour therapy uses appropriate colours to alter mood and restore harmony and balance in the body. Each colour releases different energy vibrations. The colours we choose for our walls, food, clothes and outside scenery, impact our emotional states. Sitting under a green light or a light bulb covered with green gel encourages positive thoughts. Green is said to be the colour soothing shock and pain. Blue and indigo promote healing. Red food restores energy. In general cool colours, such as blue, green, indigo and purple, help to calm painful areas and restore energy flow.

Colour	Properties	Healing uses
Red	Stimulating	Low energy
Orange	Cheering	Depression
Yellow	Helping mental detachment	Removing toxins
Green	Bringing freshness, harmony	Balancing, decreasing headaches
Blue	Calming, promoting inner reflection	Insomnia, throat problems, general healing
Indigo	Transforming, purifying	Painkiller, treating migraine and inflammations
Purple	Dignifying	Love of self, treating psychological conditions
Magenta	Letting go	Treating emotional hurts
Black	Absorbing	Self-discipline and need to hide
White	Reflecting, purity	Tonic replacing all colours
Gold	Divine power, purity (colour of the sun)	Treating depression and low energy

| Silver | Cosmic intelligence (colour of moon) | Recovery of balance, calming nerves |

Table and information summarized from Airey, *Healing Energies*, 2003, p. 36 – 39, 59.

You should select consciously or intuitively the colours fitting your healing needs the best. Of course colour therapy does not resolve issues and you should view your choice of colours as a reminder of needs to be addressed throughout the day.

WATER THERAPY TO BRING WELL-BEING

Water is essential to life. Human creation and birth are associated with water. Our bodies hold a large quantity of liquid and we die quickly if we do not get sufficient water. It is a major mistake to believe our body is a solid when it is rather a fluid always in movement. Even bones are not a solid even if they are the hardest part of the body, since calcium is eliminated and renewed every three months with food brought in to feed the body. It is not surprising that water heals. No need to go to a beach to feel better: a good warm bath, a sauna, a shower or a jacuzzi will help decrease pain.

Hydrotherapy, that uses hot, warm, cold water, ice or steam, involves several components. Drinking water eliminates waste products, flushes toxins, increases energy, decreases headaches and wrinkles on the skin. Cold sensations travel faster than pain signals to the brain and consequently prevents pain signals from easily reaching the brain. In addition, cold water stimulates endorphin release, relieves muscle spasms and decreases inflammation. It reduces migraine pain in 80 percent of cases.[30] Cold water is used in ice bags or cold packs. I like to make small rectangular bags with a soft fabric and fill them with flax seeds or rice. I keep them in the deep freezer and place one bag on my eyes to reduce headaches. Success comes from the cold temperature, slight pressure from the weight of the bag, and relaxation (if I rest on a bed with the bag on the eyes). During the summer I like to keep a pillow in the deep freezer and pull it out for bedtime to use under my neck during the night. This allows me to fall asleep with less pain.

Cold or hot water?

Warm water or steam relaxes muscle tension, decreases high blood pressure, provides increased mobility to the joints, increases the amount of endorphins in the brain and generally helps to feel better. Some say that taking a cold shower energizes the subtle energy system, seals the body's aura and stops energy from leaking out. On the other hand, flotation in warm water is said to have a deep-cleansing and balancing effect on the subtle bodies.[31]

I find cold water and icy wet compresses in general to increase muscular stiffness and pain if the temperature is too low. My personal experiences have taught me that hot pads decrease muscle pain and increase mobility, but increase sunburn pain caused by damaged nerves. It is my experience that wonderful results can be achieved by alternating very cold and fairly warm pads anywhere I feel inflammation. Everyone should try water therapy and select the best activities on an individual basis. Heat and cold are said to close the pain gates in the spinal cord[32] and they offer a strong distraction to making the brain unable to receive pain messages.

Without doubt, water therapy really does work. Drinking 8 glasses of water (about 2 litres of water) per day in addition to other liquids helps me to remove the unpleasant feeling of dry mouth caused by medication. Having a basic warm bath in the morning, even without bubbles or fancy lighting, relaxes my entire body and decreases neck pain and back pain before medication becomes fully effective. Afterwards I am ready to use the stairs in my home without stabbing pain with each step. Blowing warm air from a hair dryer on the skin or applying hot towels from the dryer sometimes decreases pain even more. Warm water brings comfort, and balances the energy because it offers an immediate feeling of well-being. The expense of a home hot tub, whirlpool or a sauna may be a tax deductible expense with a letter from a physician depending on your place of residence.

HEALING WITH FLOWERS AND HERBS

For many centuries healing systems have relied on plants containing therapeutic and medicinal properties. An estimated 25% of today's pharmaceuticals is synthesized from plants. The earliest recorded method depending on plants was found in China and dates back to about 5,000 years ago. European healers based their knowledge on Sumerian and Egyptian records as well as ancient Greek and Roman texts produced by the physicians Hippocrates, Galen,

> *Healing with flowers and herbs is as ancient as mankind, and for most of human history was the only medical option available.*
>
> Houdret, *Healing with flowers*, 2003, p. 5.

Theophrastus and Dioscorides. Flowers are said to bring universal comfort with their beauty and scent, and of course, anything offering comfort reduces pain.

Paracelsus (1493 – 1541) was a Swiss physician and alchemist who believed disease came from departure with spirituality and thought a substance called "quintessence" could heal the soul. The right essence came from a plant or a mineral and reconnected with the spirit's ability to heal. During the Renaissance it was believed that flower fragrance would protect from disease. In the early 19th century chemical preparations began to replace remedies made from plants. Edward Bach (1886 – 1936), who worked for the London Homeopathic Hospital, developed modern flower therapy. He believed that the flowers were the spirit or character of the plant. This spirit could be absorbed as an energy pattern by water, and when this liquid was taken by the one in pain, the positive components of the flowers would heal. This therapy of flowers is a close cousin to homeopathy. Bach also believed people should work on emotions, especially fear and uncertainty, in order to heal. Around 1928 he observed that certain flowers, such as impatiens and clematis, helped to heal mental states.[33]

Classification of plants

Modern herbal therapy is based on liquid herbal preparations from flowers selected by individual users wishing to restore their health by non-invasive treatment of mental-emotional conditions. Bach defined a system with the Seven Helpers, the Twelve Healers and the Nineteen Essences. The Seven Helpers which correspond to chronic conditions are: gorse, heather, oak, olive, rock water, vine and wild oat. They support the Twelve Healers that relate to the positive and negative states of 12 basic personality types and help us to find balance. The Twelve Healers are:

Negative	Essence	Positive
Restraint	Chicory	Love
Fear	Mimulus	Sympathy
Restlessness	Agrimony	Peace
Indecision	Scleranthus	Steadfastness
Indifference	Clematis	Gentleness
Weakness	Centaury	Strength
Doubt	Gentian	Understanding
Over-enthusiasm	Vervain	Tolerance
Ignorance	Cerato	Wisdom
Impatience	Impatiens	Forgiveness
Terror	Rock rose	Courage
Grief	Water violet	Joy

The following New Nineteen Essences assist in developing positive spiritual qualities: aspen, beech, cherry plum, chestnut bud, crab apple, elm, holly, honeysuckle, hornbeam, larch, mustard, pine, red chestnut, star of Bethlehem, sweet chestnut, walnut, white chestnut, wild rose, willow.

> Herbal medicine is holistic in its approach: it aims to treat the underlying causes of illness as well as the actual symptoms.
> Houdret, *Healing with herbs*, 2003, p. 5.

The Helpers, Healers and Essences receive their healing powers from the sun.[34]

Healing with flowers and herbs includes internal inhalations, teas, infusions, decoctions, tonics, tinctures, tablets, capsules and powders, and external uses such as compresses, skin creams and oils. Flowers should be picked while in bud or freshly opened, at the time when scent and taste are the strongest, and collected on a warm early morning before the sun dries them.[35]

Herbal medicine as an old therapy

Warm teas, also called tisanes or infusions, made with flowers or herbs are very common and have been used for centuries. They give a feeling of comfort in addition to the special properties attached to each flower. Teas with chamomile, known by the Greeks and the Romans, are highly recommended to relax muscles, prevent muscle spasms and reduce insomnia. Valerian was enjoyed by the Greeks and the Romans to relax and fight insomnia, and has been used for the same purpose in China for numerous centuries. This plant holds the valerian acid which acts as a sedative. Tonic teas, made from St. John's wort, sage or mugwort, restore the nervous system. Others use skullcap, vervain and wood betony, to help relax.[36] Feverfew, a member of the chrysanthemum family, is said to reduce migraines. Ginkgo tea increases blood flow to the brain and is thought to reduce tinnitus, an extremely unpleasant ringing sound in the ears. The challenge with teas is to find the appropriate dose to achieve improvement of a medical condition. Moreover, few reliable and scientific books on herbal therapy are available in English. You make tinctures by adding dried or fresh flowers to a mixture of drinkable alcohol and boiling water. The alcohol dissolves, strengthens and preserves the active ingredients found in the flowers. Tinctures are taken in small quantities. Sometimes the boiling water poured on flowers or herbs is not sufficient, harder plants must be boiled to pro-

> Flowers are conscious, intelligent forces. They have been given to us for our happiness and healing.
>
> Devi in Houdret, *Healing with flowers*, 2003, p. 22.

duce a decoction.[37]

Chamomile tea helps bring on sleep. These flowers are said to have anti-inflammatory properties. Meadowsweet tea may reduce arthritis. Dill poultices reduce joint pains. Borage tea reduces depression and anxiety. St John's wort tea and tablets are a effective anti-depressant, and interestingly a common medication called Zoloft is based on a substance accumulated in St John's wort. Juniper berries help to fight arthritis. Lemon balm tea reduces anxiety, depression and headaches. Passionflower tea relieves pain, primarily headaches and insomnia. Valerian tea reduces stress. Marjoram tea treats anxiety, insomnia, headaches, muscle pain, sprains and stiff joints. Rosemary tea eases headaches while its tincture decreases tension, depression, rheumatism and muscle pain. Comfrey leaves poultices, compresses and ointments treat inflamed muscles and strained tendons. Eating two or three leaves of feverfew decreases migraines. Lavender is the other good friend of the one with chronic pain as its tea eases headaches, stress, nervous tension and promotes sleep. California poppies are a sedative and relieve pain, anxiety and nervous tension. Primrose tea also treats anxiety and insomnia.[38] Herbs are not government regulated the way pharmaceutical medications are, and you do well to remember that some herbs are toxic. You can buy your herbs from a health store or you may want to grow them inside or outside your house.

UNDERSTANDING AROMATHERAPY

Essentials oils from herbs and flowers can hold additional beneficial properties. Aromatics, medicine and magic were interrelated in early cultures. Native Americans still burn aromatic plants like sage and sweetgrass to produce a healing, purifying smoke. In the ancient classical world in 300 B.C. Theophrastus, the Greek philosopher and Aristotle's pupil, described the properties of various oils and herbs as affecting mental power. The Ancient Greeks and Romans used aromatherapy in their daily life, however several early Christians rejected aromatherapy because it developed sensual pleasure.[39]

Aromatherapy is about the art of creating a force for wellness using essential oils, which can be inhaled or used as massage lubricant to increase well-being and distract from pain. Essential oils have an impact on mood and release healing properties as they evaporate. They can be mixed with water in a vaporizer or can be burned on a burner to add scent to a room. Essential oils can be also diluted in shampoo, shower gel or liquid soap for use in the bath water, and can be mixed with vegetable oil to be warmed and spread on the skin during massage. They are absorbed by the skin and the scent aids massage and warm baths to increase positive effects. Essential oils do not mix well with water and for this reason should be mixed with a bath product, for use on the body, since you do not want a drop of essence, floating on water, to irritate the skin.[40] With the exception of lavender oil, if used on burns or insect bites, essential oils ought not to be taken internally or used undiluted. These oils can be combined to offer several healing benefits. They improve quality of life by releasing tension, decreasing headaches, giving an emotional boost and help fight depression. Their fragrance adds pleasure to the environment. Stress forces the body to send extra blood to the muscles and increases heart rate.[41] Essential oils reduce these actions and their scent can be used at any time since oils are easily carried in a small container. You should select the oil appropriate for your activities or mental state.

This table will help to have a better understanding of healing properties offered by essential oils used to decrease pain:

Types of oils	Benefits
Orange (fruit, blossom or leaf)	Soothing effect, decreasing headaches and muscular pains, nervous tension and insomnia. Orange blossom stimulates serotonin.
Grapefruit (peel)	Reducing headaches and nervous exhaustion, decreasing muscular pains
Lime	Good tonic
Bergamot	Excellent antidepressant
Lemon	Refreshing, preventing bitterness and resentment when in pain; reducing muscular pains and stiffness
Jasmine	Relaxing, decreasing depression and muscular pains
Black pepper	Comforting, excellent for muscular aches and pain
Geranium	Antidepressant, decreasing nervous tension and exhaustion
Lavender	Reducing stress, muscular pains and stiffness. Lavender stimulates serotonin.
Rose	Anti-inflammatory, soothing muscular and nervous tension
Rosemary	Decreasing nervous exhaustion, headaches and migraines, improving blood circulation to the brain
Clary sage	Relaxing and treating depression, decreasing muscular pains and stiffness
Peppermint	Relieving headaches and muscular pains
Chamomile	Relaxing, reducing headaches and insomnia. Chamomile stimulates serotonin.

Marjoram	Decreasing headaches, muscular pains, migraines, stiffness and insomnia. Marjoram stimulates serotonin.
Ginger	Relieving muscular aches and pains
Nutmeg	Effective for muscular aches
Palmarosa	Comforting, good for headaches and nervous exhaustion
Pine	Easing muscular pain, relieving fatigue
Sandalwood	Relaxing, decreasing depression
Cedarwood	Uplifting, relaxing, soothing, preparing for meditation
Cypress	Uplifting, easing sadness, soothing
Ylang ylang	Decreasing tension, insomnia, panic attacks, anxiety and depression
Eucalyptus	Reducing muscular pains and stiffness

Source: Evans, 2003, p. 10 – 63.

I believe the queen of all essential oils is lavender. It is very healing, versatile, relaxing and promotes rest and sleep. Aromatherapy is an ancient therapy that is enjoying a resurgence of use and appreciation. This revival can be explained by the fact that aromatherapy has very few, if any, dangerous side effects if employed properly. At the same time it is an easy and affordable way to heal the body, mind and soul.

Scientists confirm the sense of smell is unique and particularly capable of evoking memories and emotions. All senses, except for smell, depend on a "filtering process in the brain" that is governed by the thalamus and "helps screen out sensory input that is nonsensical or extraneous."[42] It is important to note that smell goes directly to the brain's limbic system where memory and emotions are processed. In addition, smell is said to "cause secretion of the brain chemicals that are associated with those moods."[43] It is not surprising that aromatherapy is effective in recreating a feeling of lost well-being.

HORTICULTURAL THERAPY

We plant particular flowers and select trees because we connect with them and find happiness in closely following the seasons, patiently waiting for blooms and scents while watching growth. Plants mean something to us. Look at my garden! It retraces all of the chapters and past images of my life. The jasmine, the geraniums and lavender are reminders of the Mediterranean shore where I was born and did archaeological work. I close my eyes and the scent magically sends me back to Provence, Capri or Sicily where geraniums become bushes. These flowers have the power to open the door to my past and to lead me to other flowers and numerous other scents.

Several flowers in my garden have been selected because of their colours. I

> *Many of us have happy memories of a garden. As a sufferer of chronic pain, I believe a garden can be a powerful means to maintain happiness and to heal our body, mind and soul during a lifetime. It is a rainbow illuminating your life, a friend, a symphony, a impressionist painting or a love song, all in all an unique piece of artwork where colours are selected as carefully as a note for a musical piece, a touch of colour for a painting or a word for a poem; in addition a garden is a family photo album retracing our past and heritage, an autobiography and a mirror of ourselves. With such riches to enjoy, physical pain becomes more supportable. Such is the magic of all our gardens.*
>
> Dr. Claude M. Roberto

imagine the final results when the painting is finished and each flower is the stroke of an invisible paint brush. I avoid monotony, repetition and stiffness by mixing flowers. I play with their colours, textures, shapes, heights, sunny areas and shade, with sun and moon in the midnight part of the garden holding white flowers; and of course in Canada I challenge seasons with flowers from early May to early November. Roses and calendulas resist well into fall and they can even survive the first frost.

Gardens become part of the family, providing historical milestones. My tamarac was planted when my first daughter was born. The horse chestnut tree is as old as my second daughter. The front crabapple trees were in full bloom when she was born, and the blue delphiniums started to bloom in 1998 when I left for an overseas holidays with the children.

Of course bushes and trees also grow with the pain. How little were the rose bushes where I came back from the hospital after the car accident! Gardens are also good friends who are always faithful and available. Just like friends they need care, unconditional love and nutrition. They can't wait when they ask for water. In return for this care, they offer a healing refuge where I can escape, rest, read, relax the mind, nurture and recharge my soul, forget daily worries, reconcile with the world, be peaceful, breathe deeply, age in technicolor, meditate and enjoy nature harmony and beauty always inspiring and giving me strength to go on. I see my garden as a sacred place encouraging me to pause, slow down and continue with renewed energy.

Plants and flowers enhance the quality of life. They release negative emotions. They are a sign of harmony with nature because, when we care for them, we connect with the universe. They can heal you through gardening activities that encourage hope, increase feelings of well-being, lower blood pressure and force you to exercise in a pleasant environment. This therapy involves scents of flowers, sounds from birds and water fountains as well as it reduces stress and has an impact on our emotions. Connecting with flowers is another source of healing. It is said that gardening can produce endorphins in the same way as jogging and cycling.[44] The ones experiencing pain interested in gardens find it easier to socialize by visiting other gardeners and exchanging plants. Belonging to a group remains a viable way to heal a life. Creating beauty and nurturing the imagination bring relief from pain. Even those without artistic talents can grow flowers and develop displays of colours. Benefits from horticultural therapy are backed by scientific research.

In a healing garden everybody should be welcome. This means planters may be higher for the fragrances of flowers to be accessible to people on wheelchairs. In order to create a healing environment the garden should touch the five senses with spectrums of colours, scents, rustling grasses or chimes, aromatic herbs or flowers, like pansies, calendulas or nasturtiums, to be tasted and touched.

Up to you for a selection

During your recovery from pain and search for peace, you will examine and decide which energy therapy you prefer. Any or all of them may work for you but your challenge will be to select one or two for implementation at the right moment and to combine them, as much as possible, with conventional North American medicine if you wish and can do so. You will then consider whether you should experiment with other types of energy practices and add them to your life. You will decide which ones to keep in your programme. Your medical team should be informed as to your choices of alternative therapies. The cost of the therapy, personal preferences and positive results are all components of your choice.

We wish to end with a warning: alternative medicine can be followed for personal reasons or when our conventional medicine fails; it can be often combined with North American practices. However alternative medicine does not make miracles and certain treatments are not compatible with scientific medicine. The client does not always know the nature of herbs prescribed by Chinese physicians and these natural products may have unwanted effects if taken with non traditional medication. Sometimes a combination of different practices has no published results, therefore results and consequences are only known from following the combined therapies.

You should not use Chinese medicine to compensate for mistakes or secondary effects caused by scientific medicine because these non traditional therapies may be irreversible; in addition, Chinese physicians are trained to deal with syndromes, not with unwanted effects from modern medicine. We ought to remember alternative medicine does not quickly "fix" clients and may require additional pain as well as hard work before offering any positive results. However traditional Chinese medicine and North American scientific medicine have each a role to play and both allow in different ways to heal and reach peace with pain.

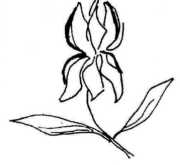

Chapter 6

CONNECTIONS

It is true that social connections help to heal and give meaning to life. At the same time people are healing agents who can improve quality of life. Unfortunately social isolation is very common among the ones in pain, especially older people who are at an even higher risk of death. Failure to grasp that human beings are interconnected leads to significant errors that cause pain and prevent healing. Pain can provide an opportunity to ask for and receive help, and thereby to connect more with people. Connection is a requirement for happiness.

> **Healing is a communal experience; it is contagious just like infection.**
> Marc Ian Barasch in Brody, 2000, p. 192.

It is not surprising then that any good pain management plan views social connections as having an important impact upon body, mind and soul. Such a plan begins with a commitment to life and healing as well as to the development of trust. A good plan is not easy to start because trust involves sharing experience with someone, which always leads to vulnerability. People who have experienced betrayal of trust may find themselves unable to share the burden, seek out solutions and ultimately heal. The challenge is to find the right people with whom to connect. The right people will provide a safe environment for sharing. Ideally these people will offer unconditional love and compassion. They become a part of our mission or purpose in life which will be defined later on. They will not judge, will not seek to impose barriers to healing, and will not accept common misconceptions attached to chronic pain.

A COMMITMENT TO HEAL

An effective pain management plan demands that we trust specific people. We do well to give priority to communicating and connecting with others, including our medical team, coworkers, partners, clients and other stakeholders, community, friends, and family. Love and intimacy are synonymous with connection and good communication. Positive relationships do not exist without love. Love breaks isolation and loving relationships are widely understood to positively affect health and longevity. The person in pain who comes to accept that he or she is lovable is able to

> The people in the east show the utmost kindness and compassion to the sick and the suffering. This has greater effect than the remedy itself. You must always have this thought of love and affection when you are visiting the ailing and afflicted.
>
> Abdu'l-Baha from Huddleston, 1996, p. 70.

heal and find peace. But love is a two way street. The person in pain does well to offer love to others because offering love brings positive healing energy in return. We believe that social ties, involving a love exchange, and connection with significant persons at home, at work and in the community play a role in healing and protecting against pain and disease.[1] The following formula takes into account the causes of pain and not just the symptoms. It is the one we will defend as the best because we see all people as connected and part of the same universe. We believe that lack of love and connection increases pain. Indeed, it may be the most important cause of pain.

Commitment to life and healing = connections + trust =vulnerability = love + intimacy = healing + fulfilling mission in life

Fear / no commitment = mistrust / cynicism = hostility = closed off = isolation = disease / pain / premature death[2]

The ones living with chronic pain must first choose the formula by establishing appropriate connections with appropriate people. Pain is complex and cannot be treated solely with connections, however, positive relationships reduce suffering. Of course you risk becoming vulnerable when you share emotions with others who learn more about you in the process. This vulnerability comes from providing confidential information to another person (when you love someone, how can you hide the dark side of your life?) and also from the risk the other person being unable or unwilling to reciprocate. It may hurt even more if the other person doesn't respond to love. However, intimacy resulting from a connection can be very healing and will help to establish a purpose in life. Mistrust and cynicism cause isolation. Isolation leads to additional pain and disease, which in turn can bring feelings of emptiness, wasted energy, and even premature death. We want to add that pain most commonly seems unfair and needless even though it forces us to seek love, healing and a purpose in life. We may easily overlook the positive consequences of our discomfort.

CONNECTIONS WITH YOUR MEDICAL TEAM

We believe that care, compassion and intimacy must be the elements which connect the client and the medical team. Interconnectedness is essential in removing the loneliness and isolation often felt by those in pain. This is especially true when the symptoms are invisible and when for this reason, compassion is not offered by others. Positive energy and peace are created in the client's life when the client feels loved and supported by the medical team. Pain decreases, healing occurs and medication becomes more effective. Information flows much better. The client should be the centre of an interconnectedness in which every professional member of the team perforce must participate. The team includes physicians and various specialists, psychologists, massage therapists, chiropractors, physiotherapists and other healthcare professionals. This team must welcome active and assertive clients who can be supported without becoming dependent. Professional qualifications are meaningless if the service provided lacks compassion. Clients know their condition best. However

> *Physicians must take down the barriers, take off the white coats and participate in the healing relationship as living beings. To do this, they must act from their own woundedness; and when they do, the effect on their patients is instantaneous.*
>
> Greenwood and Nunn, 1994, p. 242 – 243.

they do well to inform themselves of technical matters to help them make informed treatment choices.

Loving and caring

The medical team does not treat only on the body but the entire person since "our emotions are intertwined with every aspect of our physiology" and "in fact, the emotions originate as a field that flows all around and through the brain, glands, immune system, heart, and intestines, making up a complete informational network."[3] Hugging is important because it "is a moving out of isolation, and if a person can really relax into a hug, it is healing" and "any kind of physical touch, as long as the person welcomes it, is a way of moving out of isolation."[4] Recent research has shown that a lack of love and intimacy negatively impacts molecules and mechanisms. A lack of normal nurturing as children affects biological processes, can impair brain development making us more sensitive to pain and depression.[5] In infants, lack of connection can easily prove fatal.

Caring stimulates placebos and you should leave your doctor's office having experienced warm human contact.[6] Therapists generally are not trained to tell you they care for you. In fact, many therapists hold their licenses at the whim of regulating bodies that discourage their expressing how they feel towards clients. It is important therefore to analyze your feelings after visiting your care providers. You should trust your intuition to let you know whether or not your therapists are real healers who care for you.

It has been noted that many people who commit or attempt suicide while in treatment see their therapists as maintaining "a detached, analytic distance from them." Good therapists do not stay in a "detached mode" and it is certainly recognized by some that "maintaining a distance is going to make the person worse."[7] Conversely, good relationships with physicians greatly affect the effects of medication and treatment. Clients who are well connected to physicians (those even using placebos) usually feel better that the ones using large doses of medication who have poor relationships with their medical team.

Ideal therapists become the clients' agents in health care matters[8] helping them gain the best sense of being in charge of their lives and their medical conditions.[9]

I also believe therapists do well to view their clients as genuine partners in creating health and wellness. Clients should never feel alone or abandoned, and need to be in a position to make decisions regarding treatment.[10] The positive attributes of therapists must also be shared by the office staff since many interactions occur with them. It is believed that a good healing relationship between people in pain, therapists and their office staff involves care, sensitivity, empathy, trust and freedom for the clients to make decisions.[11] However it must be recognized that patients have different preferences and expectations.

You should identify your own needs and define the therapists you prefer to visit before interviewing them and deciding who will treat you. Gender preferences should be considered if applicable. Age and experience may also be factors in your decision.[12] Friends, family members and spouses should never make pressure on the person in pain to select therapists of their choice. Freedom of choice is essential in the therapeutic relationship.

Personally, I prefer therapists who, in addition to being highly skilled and technically competent, are good team players with varied backgrounds. Psychologists, massage therapists, chiropractors, physiotherapists and other health care providers are all parts of my team. I find the pain management team, including myself, has better results when everyone communicates well and actively participates. It is also important that physicians and therapists understand how chronic pain affects all aspects of life including relationships, family, career, income and hobbies.

How to build your team

The client is responsible for interviewing and identifying potential team members. Not all physicians will embrace this vision of a integrated team and may be able to meet the needs of an active client. Affinities must exist between all the team members in order to maintain a long term interconnectedness and focus on the same goal. Since pain is such a complex issue, this interconnectedness will carry on through many years, possibly even a lifetime. If you are able to talk with your therapists about non-medical events in your life and in their lives, you are well connected with your team. Clients don't ever forget those therapists who connected with them and kept them on the right track.[13]

Team members must be nonjudgmental and accept the client as he or she is. This is one of the most important components of unconditional love. Harsh judgment usually destroys the love, communication and compassion so essential to connections. This means the client should be free to test different treatments, to use alternative medical practices as well as to access narcotics, without being afraid to discuss these choices with the medical team.

Due to the high degree of specialization between health care providers, the medical team will be comprised of several members. Numerous therapists are a good tool because interaction can help decrease pain. The responsibility for establishing relationships belongs typically to the client and this is not easy to develop or maintain.

It is unrealistic to expect a clear diagnosis from your family physician because pain is so complex. Good physicians usually note concerns and symptoms before arriving at a diagnosis and prescribing treatment. They need clear information regarding the client's expectations. What do you expect from the visit? Concerns should be summarized (no more than 3 or so per visit) and prioritized because physicians do not typically have more than 15 minutes to spend with a client. It is prudent to routinely request double booking because chronic pain issues are complex and may require additional time. Time saving during visits is important: We found that bringing written notes, such as medication doses and side effects, and about three questions per visit work well. Written notes save time, in part because they free the physician from writing some information. The physician has then more time to devote to discussion with the person in pain. Clients and physicians do not typically have the same agenda. Clients look for ways to be free of pain as quickly as possible while physicians follow formal procedures and may have no quick solutions to offer. The client should feel empowered and well-informed following the visit, so clients should question what they do not understand. Physicians do well to choose non-medical terminology in order to facilitate improved communication and understanding.

No to a third party!

Sometimes it may be recommended to bring a friend or a spouse when you visit the physician. This would be especially helpful for a shy person. This is not however advisable at all if the client is able to think, hear and speak clearly. Third parties may make it very difficult for the client and the physician to connect and exchange confidential information. The conversation with three participants may easily take a turn to exclude the client if the friend or spouse is talkative or is too assertive. Relationships may be also a sorrowful subject for the client because the ones experiencing chronic pain often suffer from isolation. This painful subject may not readily be discussed in the presence of a third party and even of a spouse. In addition, if the client visits the physician with another third person, the client can become quickly a subject of conversation between the physician and the third person rather than the person in need for pain relief. Of course, in some cases, it may be useful for a client to visit a physician with a friend, if for example the client is very ill or needs additional emotional support.

How much knowledge should the client receive?

The amount of knowledge someone obtains from the library or Internet may cause other issues. If the client shows too much knowledge, the physician may be uncomfortable especially in this area where little is well known. Clients should use intuition when sharing knowledge and asking questions. Another potential conflict can arise from the use of alternate treatments the physician may recommend. Clients and physicians should agree on the type of treatments to be followed, especially in areas where various traditional and non-traditional treatments should be tried to develop a pain management plan.

Sources of conflict to avoid

A family doctor knowledgeable about the client is usually the best choice for care, however if the family physician is uncomfortable with recommendations from other healthcare providers, the client may have to select another doctor who shares affinities. Chronic pain can be

AT PEACE WITH PAIN

very frightening as is replacing a family doctor. We may not know until after a few visits whether the choice was a good one. The family physician is such a critical team member that we should take every precaution to ensure we have one who loves us and fits well with us during challenging times. Trust is essential in the relationship with a physician and for this reason, the ones with chronic pain and their physicians need to be able to function in complete harmony. Friends, family members or spouses may not agree with the selection of a therapist by the one in pain, but they should not throw a negative shadow on the therapeutic alliance between the client and the therapist. Otherwise the one in pain will not heal.

Conflict between the client and a physician may appear when, for example, the client is involved in litigation. Some physicians refuse to treat persons having experienced a car accident and this position is on the borderline with discrimination because injuries can be the same for clients in litigation and for the ones not in litigation. Therefore it is not advisable to discriminate between health care users because of their legal situation. Providing information may also lead to conflicts. The information on the medical files, such as the information in the pain diary, belongs to the client, but the personal notes and interpretations belong to the doctor and his/her corporation. When third parties such as insurance carriers and lawyers require medical documentation, the client must agree in writing to the release of it by the physician. However, the client has no control over the type or interpretation of information the doctor will provide. Trust between the client and the physician is even more essential in this type of situation. Ideally the physician should inform the client as to the nature of reports being provided. If this does not happen, the client may then receive a copy of this information from the lawyer. Overall, it is desirable for the client to receive the information directly from the doctor. This is also better for the client wishing to coordinate other activities attached to healing.

Another potential conflict may arise from the expectation of truth from the family doctor. Clients often expect to be told they will heal quickly and may expect physicians to give them a magic solution for healing. There is no magic, doctors do not know all the answers. In the uncertain field of pain, do we need someone to be positive and give us hope? Are we able to handle truth? What is truth in an area as complex as pain? Since there are so few standard treatments with chronic pain, it is often impossible to predict the final outcome with any certainty. Nothing is certain because pain remains a major puzzle. However the quality of information received from the physician will have a major impact on the client's emotions and health. If the physician and client relationship is positive, it will be easier for the client to deal with truth or any versions of it. In relationships where the client feels loved and supported, he or she will have more energy to heal and fight pain. The client will be less anxious and will trust the physician if he or she feels loved by the physician.

We believe physicians do well to honestly describe different possible realistic outcomes, knowing that the results are usually unpredictable. Doctors are only able to describe outcomes experienced by other clients for specific treatments. As no two clients are identical, physicians are not generally able to predict if the same results will occur in seemingly similar situations. Not everyone heals in the same way given the same medication, treatments and pain management plans.[14]

The physician also needs to reassure the client that he or she is not alone in this struggle against pain. It feels so good to hear from the physician "We will win and make peace with pain" or "We will manage your pain together" because these words reassure and help send away feelings of loneliness and isolation. Intimate exchange of information is also facilitated because the client feels connected with the doctor and does not feel blamed, judged or embarrassed when explaining personal issues. Good communication, support, trust, compassion and love in the physician – client relationship are essential, especially if family and communities do not always understand the nature of pain.

Being honest and speaking openly about controversial treatments help to assess the resiliency of the doctor – client relationship. Through courageous efforts in service of bearing witness to the truth, clients come to know or understand when it is time to end a relationship and look for another physician. When truth fails to resolve tension, it becomes obvious that the healing relationship has become too difficult to maintain.[15]

The physicians' gender may have an interesting impact on the doctor – client relationship. Some people have difficulty connecting with physicians other than those of their own gender and so seek medical care accordingly. Physicians who have personal experience dealing with pain often are more able to provide care to the ones with chronic pain, and connect through the shared experience. We believe it helps the physician to communicate with the client when both sides have a personal knowledge of pain. However this experience is not crucial. We need knowledgeable and well trained doctors who are able to love, care, reduce distance, show compassion and practice empathy. These characteristics are more important than personal experience with pain. Unfortunately they are difficult to communicate in the traditional academic environment. Expressed compassion facilitates the therapeutic alliance which is essential in managing pain.[16] The relationship between caregiver and the one in pain is a key element in healing and surprisingly a large number of clients taking placebos recover when they feel loved and respected by their physicians.

The many partners of a medical team

For reasons more related to history than to logic and/or skill, the family medical doctor is a central figure among healthcare providers. However he or she does well to freely share roles and responsibilities with other healers. Psychologists, chiropractors, massage therapists, physiotherapists and nurses, all hold an important place in a complete pain management plan. The client selects members of the team, and coordinates the services they offer. A therapeutic alliance exists between the client and each team member. We believe all these relationships are best built on the model we proposed for the alliance between the client and the family doctor.

CONNECTIONS AT THE WORKPLACE

Connections at work are often difficult and possible only in certain work environments. Colleagues may be concerned about work performance either because they genuinely care for us or because they believe we are unable to achieve high performance (this is usually due to fully justified but unacceptable absences which create performance concerns). Most colleagues will watch without asking questions, while others will wonder how long we will be able to continue to work. Toxic work places where pain grows as soon as you enter the building are not rare at all. Quite the opposite, in fact.

The threat of bullying

Bullying is well known to occur among children, but it also happens between adults at work. Workplace bullying is a common issue for people who have chronic pain. Bullying creates imbalance or abuse of power by setting one individual or a group towards another. The goal of the bully is to overpower the targeted person emotionally, physically, socially or verbally.[17] The disabled are more vulnerable to bullying, and while bullying often exists between peers, it is more often superiors or managers who are the perpetrators. This type of abuse is found mainly in workplaces thriving on authoritarian rule where upper-level managers act in superior, threatening ways that put at risk the well-being of all staff.[18] Workers need to know they are protected against this type of abuse by unions, labour standards and human rights legislation.

Authors identified the following five major types of workplace bullying: threats to professional status (public humiliation or/and disregarding or minimizing opinions), threats to personal standing (name-calling, intimidation or rumor mongering), isolation (withholding of information and shunning), overwork (unreasonable deadlines and frequent unnecessary interruptions), and destabilization (failure to receive credit for work and lessening of responsibilities).[19] People with chronic pain may be more fragile than healthy staff and bullying makes it even more difficult to manage pain.

It can be challenging to find workplaces where coworkers and management love you, do not force you to work
defensively, are not mean, see the soul beyond the body
and invite you to be part of the business decision making
process. Trust is possible in these places and some healing will come from them. If you look carefully, you may
find happy places where people smile at you, wait for the
answer when they ask you how you feel and, all in all, care
for you.

We find such paradise in places where compassion, care,
spirituality and faith are present and where employees have
an opportunity to relax, use intuition, heal their wounds,
work as a team, grow, produce and develop at their own
speed. In these places, kindness is a recognized virtue and
employees love each other even when their company faces
the stressors common to all businesses. These places are
associated with high road work which characterizes positions answering the needs of the soul and driven by moral
values, not just by financial profit.

Positions attached to challenging and difficult issues,
such as financial investments or delivery of justice, can
also belong to this category of high road work.[20] Even legal
firms, known for being highly competitive, can protect
human rights, care for clients, seek justice based on truth,
a condition to suit the soul, and may not see income as
their top priority. It is possible to find such high moral
standards in many professions because the values you
follow and the love you put in your profession can often
change your job (by definition, a low road activity) into
high road work. This "soft" approach may be less profit-
able to the business in the short term, but final profits will
ultimately increase.

Job or work?

We should distinguish between a job and work. A job satisfies financial needs. In contrast, work satisfies emotional, cognitive, and spiritual needs. Work may provide large amounts of money or it may not. Work may give meaning to life and provide happiness. It may be especially meaningful to those who face physical or mental challenges. People with chronic pain do well to seek work rather than a job. In an ideal world, job and work would be the same, and would at once provide financial, emotional, mental and spiritual security. Unfortunately life rarely presents ideal conditions. In the real world jobs far outnumber opportunities for work.[21] In the context of employment, trust and healing are too often impossible to find.

A healing workplace

A major challenge, faced by people with special needs such as chronic pain, lies in the fact that society judges people by occupational and financial status. This relates to occupational stress. The more money and more stress people receive, the higher their position is valued in the world and the higher is the respect received from others. This remains the traditional perception.

Money = worth = success = dignity = place in the sun = place in society

Pain = disability = unemployment = perception of laziness = drain or weight on working force

We believe it is possible for those with chronic pain to find a place in a working environment resulting in success and dignity, allowing interdependence, connection, trust and healing.[22] This is not easy. Pursuing personal adaptation with fear is one prerequisite. Workplaces where competition and revenue generation are the primary goal of business will never accommodate anyone who has special needs. In these places, healing is impossible. Other places, where individuals perform jobs with heavy physical demands, are also not recommended for the ones in chronic pain. Workers who are less well educated and lack transferable skills, and those who are older and in a lower socioeconomic class are seen to be more vulnerable in the workplace. It can be extremely difficult to change traditional beliefs and misconceptions in a traditional workplace, especially if they are supported by management having no knowledge and/or trust in chronic pain treatment.

We believe it is possible to have chronic pain and to maintain function if several elements are present in the workplace. When the opportunity is given to assess skills (or have them assessed professionally), to offer them as part of given love, and to receive in return supportive feedback, trust, and the possibility to grow, people with chronic conditions continue to function. Healing flows then as a natural consequence. Several people have experienced chronic pain, reached their goals and made the world a better place. We can name the French impressionist painter Renoir, the German writer Goethe, St Francis of Assisi, Ste Marguerite d'Youville who founded the Sisters of Charity in Canada, the health care futurist Florence Nightingale, the actress Audrey Hepburn, the famous dancer Rudolph Noureïev who created a foundation to help people having AIDS and the artist Matisse who asked a family member to sign on his paintings his name because of his disabilities. In spite of their chronic pain, these individuals had a positive impact on many other people.

Persons with chronic pain should remember that pain and suffering are not synonyms. Suffering may be avoided by not engaging in fruitless and negative activities such as complaining that drains energy from others and makes a victim of the person in pain. This should be avoided. One cannot embrace a victim role and grow their soul at the same time. Activities suiting the needs of the soul are important because taking care of the mind and the soul are essential parts of any effective long term pain management plan. Also to be avoided is staying home alone without a passion in life, because doing so will usually increase the dysphoria often associated with chronic pain, such as fear, anxiety, depression, emptiness, resentment, worthlessness, and rejection. Remaining home bound usually reduces income, making it difficult to finance medical care. It eliminates pleasant distractions associated with work outside the home. It also becomes more difficult to connect and heal. Although we did not choose to be in pain, we can choose how to respond to our situation and how to negotiate peace with pain. If we have only a job, it may be beneficial to perform volunteer work. One must be mindful that this commitment which must be honored, increases our load. However holding only a job is generally unsatisfactory and thus painful. One does well to keep in mind that volunteers contribute to an organization as much as paid workers, and that volunteer work can be even more demanding than a salaried job, although significantly more rewarding.

What are your personal needs? What are the conditions that will ensure you a good workplace? You consider these questions and find answers before looking for a position. The first step is to focus on personal and transferable skills and assets and to evaluate your reasons for working. If it is for financial gain, try to obtain a lucrative job, and thus increase your satisfaction. If work does not completely satisfy you, having a job will at least allow time to pursue satisfactory goals. These goals will always be attached to achieving a purpose in life and to healing.

When the nature of the occupation is decided according to financial needs, it is essential to review positive and realistic goals, possibly unrelated to the job. Reaching such goals brings the kinds of joy required to develop high quality in life. Examples of these goals are playing with children, spending time with family and friends, exercising and getting fresh air, pursuing a meaningful hobby inside or outside the home, developing new relationships with nurturing people, joining a support group, visiting a therapist or undertaking any activities that will introduce a healing element in your life. You then prioritize your goals and you focus on the top ones, allowing trust, love and healing, if they are compatible with maintaining a job. Activities attached to positive goals are important to healing, although they may be unrelated to financial need. It is sometimes useful to visualize the outcomes because this exercise will give you additional motivation to attain results essential to the goals and to healing. Also, everything that has ever been achieved has been visualized beforehand.

Fortunately, in some cases it is possible to combine work with a job. The key is to find and maintain meaningful work that promotes connections and gives healing energy. This meaningful work is often called the high road and includes activities we enjoy, regardless of how much it pays, how much status is involved and what friends and family think.[23] We do these activities because we feel better when we have them in our lives, and we recognize them also when time flies by and we do not feel chronic pain any more. These activities are passions and they have a healing power. Remember that passions give energy and are conditions for success.

Follow your passions!

Passions help average people to become champions and help us to go beyond our own limits. If we do not like what we do and if we have no relationships, we will not have the energy to manage pain and experience healing. So, please develop a passion in life, develop an activity with which you identify, that will be of service to others and to you because it will give you the feeling that you are a valuable human being. These are the activities where you connect with people. How are passions to be recognized? Passions have this characteristic: they involve the heart in loving. This could be love for children, animals, flowers, could involve spirituality, or painting, writing or playing a musical instrument. Usually passions add beauty to the world and this quality increases their value even more. Passions allow you to meet people you can trust and who will help you to heal. Passions take you into a beautiful world where you forget your pain.

To be successful at a job and/or at work, we must be in a positive work environment which does not destroy self-esteem, where we feel safe, where our passions are allowed, where we have a chance to balance work and other needs (such as medical appointments, and family),

> Passions lead you to fulfill your mission or purpose in life. They take you into an extraordinary space out of the ordinary and out of chronic pain.
>
> Dr. Claude M. Roberto

if possible where we participate in decision-making and are able to keep a sense of humor.

The right organization for your needs

People with chronic pain feel better in organizations where there is no culture of abuse, where co-workers love you, where it is possible to open emails without fear, where no one is mean and managers have good people skills. Look for a workplace where employees participate in developing their organization's mission statement, where appreciation is part of daily life and employees are not taken for granted. Several employers believe that employees with a long term illness or disability are going to stay at one place for the rest of their life because no other employer will be interested in hiring someone with an illness and disability. This is just a misconception and it is wrong. Do avoid workplaces where a negative environment pumps away energy, unless they pay you a phenomenal salary and allow you to develop a passion and some high road work on the side.

You need a workplace where you feel loved, trusted and accepted without being forced to hide your pain. It is good to be in a warm and flexible place allowing you to maintain your energy and find answers to your healing needs. Energy and well-being decrease quickly in negative work environments where feelings are suppressed and you must walk with your back to the walls avoiding the knives being thrown at you. As noted by Ornish "with constant vigilance comes chronic stress and often enormous suffering."[24] We could debate whether it is better to love the beneficial work or your co-workers. Our answer will be that both doing, good and high road people, are connected. If we meet high road people, they will introduce us to beneficial work. These people are easy to recognize because they offer us unconditional love, borne of their passion for what they do.

People living with chronic pain and degenerative diseases are the people who smile to you on the phone or in person at the reception (don't forget pain is invisible), help you to hang your coat or call a taxi, make you feel welcome, look after your family or prepare wonderful meals in the local school cafeteria. They can also be teachers, medical doctors, lawyers, architects, accountants or financial advisors. These people feel better in a work environment where they have the opportunity to combine a job with meaningful work bringing joy and beauty to the world. Some of them perform ordinary tasks in a safe environment, and are appreciated by extraordinarily caring managers whom they trust and who help them grow and heal. These employees can also be appreciated by colleagues, visitors and clients who connect with them. When they receive love and support from people around them, they produce more and at a higher quality because they are happy, and this inspires love and passion for the work. Their attitude of service and unconditional love transforms ordinary activities into extraordinary and spiritual ones evoking healing all around them.[25] They know they are part of a whole, and even of the universe. Here we can make a parallel with a quote from Albert Einstein who believed that "our task must be to free ourselves from a prison by widening our circle of compassion to embrace all living beings and all of nature."[26]

Most employees, such as the ones we meet in every day life, will never receive a Nobel Prize. This is not a concern. Dr. George Wald, a Harvard biologist and winner of the Nobel Prize, wrote: "What one really needs is not Nobel laureates but love. How do you think one gets to be a Nobel laureate? Wanting love, that's how. Wanting it so bad one works all the time and ends up a Nobel laureate. It's a consolation prize. What matters is love."[27]

People with pain are easily hurt. Many are not conditioned to receive care. They tend to experience things more deeply than others and feel guilt for no reason. This implies very high levels of excitement, joy or depression, and emotional needs are higher among people in pain. Anything said the wrong way, can hurt even when intentions are the best. Have you ever heard something like "Why don't you get a disability pension and spend more time with your children?" or "If I were you, I would stay at home." These words can take on an upsetting meaning for the ones in pain. According to my personal experience, any lies, even the ones told with the best intentions, are detected quickly because people in pain have radar to detect them. It is therefore important to have co-workers with good people skills and managers or partners able to see the person beyond pain and illnesses.

Work becomes more meaningful if you have co-workers who give you unconditional support and if you are able to develop relationships or connections with them. This is based on my experience with pain. People with chronic pain often have deeper relationships than most people, but usually these connections occur with only a few persons because of having less free time for social life. They may also have huge emotional needs that can frighten most other people. But don't worry, in relationships, quality is more important than quantity.

Intuition, relaxation and beauty as useful tools

It is important to have the opportunity to use intuition[28] and find time to relax at work so that pain can be avoided as much as possible during the day. Intuition provides additional power to make decisions, simplify work, allow people to find peaceful solutions to issues, and helps to lead and to bring serenity. Intuition is a natural skill originating from an intelligence level deeper than the one coming from our conscious state. We register information without knowing it and intuition helps us to retrieve this data when needed.[29]

Relaxation does not have to be complicated. We do well to practice the ability to take a break and do some deep breathing or stretching movements. Visualization is a wonderful tool to use at work since no one knows what you imagine and visualize. The letters and numbers on your computer screen could magically become an image with mountains or with the sea, it could be summer holidays, it could be a world without pain, it could be the face of a loved one. It could be our own private space that allows us to smile even in the most difficult situations. Visualization helps one escape from negativity and disconnect from a painful reality. It is a very good relaxation exercise if you have a job. You can practice almost anywhere.

Anything adding beauty to the working place increases healing. I believe spring flowers in winter bring hope, roses offer a touch of love and elegance, lilies and daisies add spirituality. Teddy bears on a desk or a chair remind us of the importance of hugging that promotes healing. It is not surprising that they became the logo of the Chronic Pain Association of Canada a few years ago!

A continuing challenge at work, for all employees and especially those with chronic pain, is the struggle

> **The pain passes but the beauty remains.**
>
> Auguste Renoir, French impressionist painter who suffered from arthritis and whose hands were distorted by the illness, from Dillard, 2002, p. 158.

to accomplish more in less time. People who have pain

issues can do well at this because they learn how to give the appropriate size to issues. They know how healing is important, and, for example, if a project does not turn out the way it should be, their intuition will help them to find solutions. They know also that if they do not manage their disappointment and become upset, their pain will increase and become more difficult to manage. Therefore many people in pain immediately seek solutions. Pain tells them what is important and what is not. Pain taught them that intimacy and connections will help them to solve many work related issues.

Not every workplace is able to accommodate people with chronic pain. Things such as being able to move and change position are priorities. Flex time is useful to help combine work with other demands, such as health and family. Work involving creativity or distraction, as service, forces one to send pain to the back of the mind. Organizational structures in the shape of a pyramid, with a boss on the top and a hierarchy of senior managers, with emphasis on authority, and not allowing creativity, trust and compassion, do not work at all for employees with chronic pain. In my experience these structures cause fear and anxiety. They have no place for trust, intuition and creativity. In fact I believe they do not work for anyone. A horizontal structure or a team where everyone is considered important and interdependent, and has a chance to be part of the decision making process, often works much better. Positions allowing passions, research, learning, interdependence and creativity, suited to the ones in pain, include places with artists, writers, healers, activists of any nature (health, education, human rights, animal rights,..), historians, sociologists and in general any professions in the arts, social studies, community work and other humanities or positions attached to a cause or vision. Being able to establish deadlines and control demands may be also requirements. However positions, within sciences or in finance, may accommodate people with pain if they contain the appropriate ingredients. It is therefore important to find the right structure, type of work, leadership and management styles, partners and procedures.

A low level of stress at work is not the only pathway to a positive work environment for at least two reasons. One, an acceptable level of stress is a subjective judgment; and two, passion, which is the key element to success, rarely is associated with low levels of stress. Rather than to look for a reduced stress environment it is important to engage in an activity, paid or unpaid, which we believe to be meaningful and beneficial to us and to others, and in line with our values and needs. This type of position will facilitate trust and connection, energy to heal and ultimately succeed because passion and love produce healing and growing energy. It contributes to our ability to tolerate necessary stresses connected to the job.

COMMUNITY CONNECTIONS

Give and receive! Doing volunteer work and helping others allow the ones in pain to heal faster and live longer. Health benefits come from the joy of helping. "Anything that helps us freely choose to transcend the boundaries of separateness is joyful." Some volunteers even report experiences similar to a "runner's high" perhaps related to sudden bursts of endorphins at a physiological level.[30] Endorphins decrease pain. Volunteers live longer and feel better. Social and religious relationships can also be important parts of a pain management plan. The ones in pain who have a strong network of friends, and are supported by family and community find it easier to manage pain. These relationships help to provide meaning in life and can also offer potential volunteer work opportunities.

Sharing personal matters with community members may be scary but it is an excellent means to develop intimacy with a few selected neighbors. Intimacy is an efficient way to rediscover the right path in life and decreases pain through sharing with others. When the pain is divided into several smaller pieces, we are no longer the only ones to feel its impact. Our difficulties become lighter.

Lack of social integration is believed to increase pain and suicide. Suicide is often associated with physical pain and integration reduces this pain. Communities become reassuring as they offer the possibility of integration and increase energy levels. There are many kinds of communities. Some are based on hobbies or interests, on culture, on place of residence, professional associations, spirituality and religious beliefs. Each community has the potential to offer healing by sharing the pain when we remove the mask covering this pain. The key element here is to find a caring, safe and compassionate community connected with our life in a meaningful manner.

It remains that many people find it difficult to develop connectedness to others. Depression adds to this challenge and chronic pain. Traditional ways to connect include telephoning friends, relatives and acquaintances, walking a pet and talking with other pet owners, and joining an interest group or support group.

Good relationships provide love and distraction to people in pain. They may involve connecting with various age groups and different cultures. One of us, president of a local school parents' association, established a partnership with a senior citizens' home located on the other side of the street. Children paraded for them on Halloween Day, sang at Christmas, played recorders and visited them on special occasions. The seniors attended concerts and displays at the school, and volunteered as story tellers and judges for science fairs. The results of this partnership were outstanding. When the seniors crossed the street, they temporarily forgot their aches and pains and had the opportunity to get a multitude of "grandchildren" who loved them. The smiles on their faces, when they were with children, were very touching. We have already reported how hugs are important in a pain management plan. From our personal experiences people in pain and the dying need hugs and ask for touching. This increases peace, reduces the fear of dying and, consequently, decreases pain. During the ultimate phase of life, physical pain and pain coming from lack of touching, are difficult to separate. Our personal experiences with people in palliative care taught us how a simple visit or act of compassion can decrease physical pain, increase the will to live and extend life. Good connections involve giving and receiving freely. People with chronic pain receive hugs and should also give hugs and share the love they receive throughout pain.

Communities and friends are also important because they can act as family substitutes. They are relatives who are chosen if family is unavailable. Communities can add a larger dimension to families and foster interdependence. They offer assistance when needed and may help fulfill our purpose in life. What a relief it can be to someone in pain to live in a nice and friendly community! A young mother can find assistance in the community to care for children if time is needed to manage her own pain. Children in pain often find friends within the community to offer them distractions and opportunities for play.

In December 2004 the Southern Asia tsunami destroyed entire communities and the rest of the world offered support to the survivors. The world became a large community offering hope and recovery.

Ordinary activities to bring healing

Good communities function as support groups and families. They promote personal and emotional safety and serve as pillows to reduce the hard impact of isolation, loneliness and aloneness causing additional pain. They offer kindness and generally make the community a better place to live. In our neighborhood in Edmonton, people in hospitals receive visits from community members offering their help. When a mother is in the hospital, other mothers look after her children by taking them to school and caring for them. The local school parent council, community league and a few churches coordinate the organization of these activities. In this same area, families gather in winter for Friday evening skating and volunteer serve hot chocolate and supervise children if parents are unable to attend. Skating is the method of connecting. During these Friday evenings, decisions are made regarding programs offered at the local school, everybody shares news and those in pain have the opportunity to discuss with others, some of them being healthcare professionals, their personal situations.

The number of projects keeps growing. One family now invites those having an interest in sacred music to sing on Friday night; another family started to work on developing a sensory and healing garden in the community league yard. These projects provide hope and support to the ones in pain living in the area.

Divide the pain with others!

Good support groups associated with pain, encourage people to share their stories. The groups should ensure they do not facilitate members becoming victims. Support group members should feel loved and connected to other members. One of the main benefits received from a support group is to be surrounded by people who care. This increases the quality of life and helps to reverse some effects of pain. It makes information easier to obtain, develops new ideas and sets goals. A support group can be "the ideal story workshop for people trying to make sense of and come to terms with a serious chronic illness." It is believed also to "stimulate the inner pharmacy" which means to offer greater resistance to pain.[31]

However some people seem to resist healing when joining a support group. This may be due to the concept

> The worst part of holding the memories is not the pain. It's the loneliness of it. Memories need to be shared.
>
> Lowry, 1993, p. 154.

of "woundology" occurring when people are unable to get beyond the limitations the wounds impose and allow the wounds live their life for them. This can be caused by a fear of identity loss and of loneliness. Support groups do well to not reinforce these feelings and to encourage members to heal rather than to remain wounded.[32] When an effective group cares for its members, it is able to balance different needs stemming from members, and reinforces the ownership of individual health. You can heal with such a group. Of course your family, including your spouse, may see a support group as a threat because your family will share quality time with your group. Your friends in the support group will also have an impact not always welcome by your family if your family wants to control your life.

In addition, communication is not always easy within a support group. People who find groups and communities helpful are often individuals willing to share their pain experience with others and demolish defensive walls within this setting. Otherwise, peace with pain may be impossible to achieve.

CONNECTIONS WITH SIGNIFICANT OTHERS

Lack of love and presence of personal issues in families are commonly known to be major obstacles to healing and happiness. These factors make recovery more difficult. On the other hand good harmony promotes comfort and security. It is fairly common knowledge that good relationships with parents, relatives and friends are essential conditions for children and teenagers to feel good about themselves.[33] People with chronic pain not residing in loving homes can experience benefits from a relationship with a good spouse if this relationship does not include deficiencies found in childhood.[34] To be in a loving relationship of some type is an essential component of pain management because pain needs to be understood, supported and valued. Intimacy with another person can be viewed as a "fusion" into another person. This promotes sharing and the will to create.[35] We have already mentioned that sharing and creativity help to reduce pain. It is very important to connect with the appropriate individuals who must be able to care, listen, share, be positive, compassionate and committed to the relationship. Unconditional love is the key element in the heart of significant partners for healing to occur. The quality of the relationship is more important than the quantity of it. In return for care and support, the ones in pain can provide unconditional love, and both actions, to give and receive, help to reduce chronic pain.

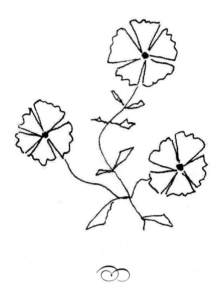

SPIRITUALITY TO HEAL

Spirituality is now scientifically recognized as an important factor in healing. Pain can put us in touch with spirituality because it is not only solved by science and, if impossible to manage, may lead to death. Pain also has a connection to the unknown because of its numerous and complex components that remain poorly understood. A sense of the meaning of life and/or help from a superior force becomes essential. Pain has an impact on the body and also on other areas, such as the mind and the soul. It is not surprising that healing a life involves healing the soul. Remember that meditation, prayer, being close to nature, and creating

beauty are means to reach out to the soul. Even gardening and planting flowers can helps heal the soul because
flowers improve life and bring beauty and magnificence.
Flowers are a sign of harmony with nature and when we
connect with growing plants, when we nurture them, we
feel in harmony with the universe.

Religion is now starting to be scientifically studied as
a healing force, possibly because religion and science are
two different fields. According to our experience, religion
can offer health advantages to those who either regularly
attend a church or who are members of a religious organization. We have seen how prayer can heal people quickly and reduce pain. More than 1 200 studies have been
published on the effects of spirituality on health. Much
of this research, identified as Frontier Medicine, has been
conducted over the last decade. According to the Nuclear
Medicine Clinic at the University of Pennsylvania, praying
is excellent for healing. A research team from this institution studied brain images of people during meditation.
These pictures revealed that the hypothalamus becomes
more active at this time. This is interesting because chemical factors originating in the hypothalamus regulate the
important stress-managing hormone cortisol.[36] The mechanism through which religion heals has not yet been
detailed. Perhaps the ones in pain get a "theological sense
of meaning" or perhaps they receive "the elements of regu-
lation of behavior within religious groups" or, maybe they
benefit from "the social contacts, relationships, and activities that go along with involvement in religious activities
and the sense of purpose that people derive from these."
Most probably people in pain get benefits from all these
healing elements.[37]

It is also believed that all relationships can be spiritual in nature because through bridging the inner life to outer life through relationships, there is some healing.[38] Prayers, even at a distance, are generally reported as improving pain and positively effecting an illness, but many people use both medications and prayers. Therefore it is difficult to separate the benefits from medication from the advantages offered by prayers. Someone in pain receiving love or offering love is transformed spiritually because love and spirituality are connected. It is again difficult, even maybe impossible, to separate the benefits from love from those offered by spirituality. However good communications, empathy and compassion or communion with someone in pain are undoubtedly spiritual activities decreasing pain. Meditation, another spiritual activity (approached in another chapter), is also a spiritual practice or tool to manage pain.

Herbert Benson was one of the first to study the effects of the mind on the body. Founder of the Mind/Body Medical Institute in Boston and teacher of medicine at Harvard University, he believes the positive benefits offered by spirituality have a scientific explanation. Prayers accompany a series of antistress physiological changes, such as slowing respiration, and have positive effects on the mind and body. Meditation may provide the same results. The belief of protection by a supreme force and connection with others by prayer can be comforting. Comfort and serenity help to reduce stress and pain. Almost one half of U.S. medical schools now present classes on health and spirituality. According to Benson, 90% of physician visits are related to stress which causes pain and which is not treated by current medical practices. Traditional medicine has little or no impact on care to the mind and the soul. Frontier Medicine will most probably become a major challenge for medicine in the third millennium.[39]

It is possible for people to manage their pain and heal, however it is understandable that many fail to do so. Some common attitudes, beliefs and emotions tend to cause isolation and prevent healing. We must not harshly judge people who may never have enjoyed the opportunity to trust, find unconditional love and discover a purpose in life. Some simply abandon the path to healing, or fail to recognize it. Pain is said to be a symptom used to discover medical issues and possibly other issues. Yes, pain can offer a chance to redirect life, trust other people and find intimacy before healing. Yes, pain can be an agent of transformation, however it is almost never experienced as a gift, or as sent by God to offer us a chance to become heroic.[40] Suffering will not likely improve any human beings because it is widely viewed as meaningless, needless, stupid and largely unfair. In fact, suffering may be the result of holding the view that the experience of pain lacks meaning and/or purpose.

PURPOSE IN LIFE

In order to heal, people who have chronic pain do well to develop and maintain a purpose in life. They should receive love and return it to others by pursuing their purpose in life. This is another way to heal. A purpose in life, also known as mission or vision, is usually connected to using your dreams and skills to create something you like, something good and important for ourselves and for others.[41] It usually is seen as the reason for being in the universe. Sharing our purpose with others is an act of kindness bringing us closer to others and allowing better connectedness. A mission is often invisible to the human eye even when the results are tangible. It may involve volunteer or paid work, or something learned from suffering. It is about doing or producing something often with limited difficulty when others consider the same activity to be almost impossible. It is commonly attached to passions and love, because passions help to go beyond our limits and love is essential to life. If love is not the purpose in life, the purpose will likely hold a good

> There is nothing in the world ... that would so effectively help one to survive even the worst conditions as the knowledge that there is meaning in one's life ... man's main concern is not to pursue pleasure or avoid pain but rather to see a meaning in his life.
>
> Viktor Frankl, German psychologist who survived life in a concentration camp, cited by Lynch, 2003, p. 65.

amount of love. A mission is a goal in life which may make it easier to live with and manage pain. When we work towards fulfilling our purpose, our suffering from pain is reduced. Energy returns and we enjoy achieving something positive for other humans in the universe. Everyone benefits because we are all part of this universe. A mission is both our reason and our method for healing and being at peace with pain. It allows for creativity and may form the key component of a bargain with pain. For example the German writer Goethe who lived with intense gout pain reported the only way for him to reduce his pain was to write for hours in his attic.[42]

> To value the ordinary can be healing and extraordinary.
>
> Dr. Claude M. Roberto and Dr. Paul S. Sussman

A satisfactory life depends on whether or not we follow our mission and are willing to be guided by passion and intuition, develop compassion and unconditional love, make decisions and be at peace.[43] Our purpose in life also requires to love what we do, increase our level of energy, and select the right direction. It forces us to focus our energy in a primary direction towards achieving our mission. Please be aware that a purpose may appear in a dream, during meditation, visualization or conversation at any time of the day or night.

Guiding signs

How can we find a purpose which will suit the needs of others and also meet the needs of our soul? How do we recognize a purpose in life among the numerous demands and activities placed upon us?

We must pay careful attention to hints or signals we receive on the direction to follow or decisions to be taken. These hints are sent to us by a force within the universe, or from God or a superior being that always will take a form we can accept. They are a sort of interior voice which can change an entire life when we put the direction into action. If it occurs one time, it may be a coincidence, however if there is a pattern (because the same or parallel signs occur repeatedly), we should solve the puzzle and attempt to discover its nature.

Signs may make purpose known by evoking fresh attention to words we have already heard, moments we seem to repeat, places we believe we have already visited and people we feel we have already met. Signs also come to us by hearing what people tell us, examining the people around us and by noting articles we find when we open a maga-

> Creativity is our natural skill giving a shape to our energy; it is the secret allowing you to have the life you want.
>
> Translated by the authors from Adrienne, 1999, p. 263 – 264.

zine[44]. These signs can help to define a purpose in life, and are sometimes referred to as synchronicity, providence or coincidence. They can be magical and helpful, and can occur apparently by chance to give us exactly what we need at the moment we need it. Signs may appear to be of little importance, but they are guides. They can offer solutions to many obstacles or worries we hide in our mind. These signs often come to us from people we meet during regular activities.[45] Did you ever phone someone exactly when this person was thinking about you? This is an example of synchronicity.

We all hide the information necessary to find our mission in life, with the starting using synchronicity to extract this information. I believe people are interdependent and solutions coming from collectivity have better results if individuals wish to feel good and succeed. Synchronicity will develop in relationship with other people with positive energy. Attraction is a type of sign. Who are the people who attract you or who are attracted by you? What could you do with them if a hint suggests that a connection would be positive? We should also remember that souls are said to be attracted by the souls of people having the same energy level as our own.

Another type of message is the feeling we have met someone previously. However we are unable to recall the name and the circumstance. The impression of *déjà-vu* is also a sign. Signs can be better recognized if we observe and love others, if we close our eyes and deeply breathe or we decide to spend some time alone. Affinities found in other people are a sign a connection should be established. Teamwork based on such an affinity can be a major success. In order to predict whether a new relationship, emotional or work related, will promote healing, it is best to form any type of affinity with this person. A few months ago, I visited a medical office. The color of the walls were the same as in our home and even the decorations and furniture were very close or identical. These are signs that a relationship with this therapist will likely be a strong one. This connection could be linked to a purpose in life. Dreams, silence or watching clouds often offer keys to hidden information which can be used in identifying a mission.[46] Sometimes even physical pain offers a clue to the right path. Headaches may try to teach us something and be a sign. It is possible to develop a dialogue with our body during the process of identifying our mission.

Intuition helps us to better understand the signs originating from a level of intelligence deeper than our conscience.[47] People who have chronic pain tend to develop their intuitions quickly because they pay attention to their bodies and minds. The way they feel in a given situation, can be a sign. Do you become relaxed just by fixing a few images? Or does pain increase while talking to someone? If pain increases, it is a sign this person will be unable to assist in any healing. When a purpose is found, we can prepare an action plan and begin healing while we conduct activities attached to the plan.[48] Energy and creativity increase when one concentrates on the present without having preconceived ideas. We see intention followed by energy. It is the force directing us and pushing us to achieve results.[49] We should not have to struggle to achieve our mission if this one is the one for us. It should not be difficult to find a purpose in life. If you are involved in an activity where you lose track of time and use specific skills, most probably you are working towards your mission. If you are worried, negative, stressed or angry, lose energy and produce negative results, you are straying away from your mission. Your environment impacts your purpose and you should change it if it damages your intention and energy. We should also keep in mind that if we are able to accept a greater force, such as a divine power, we may be at peace with pain sooner.

THE ESSENTIAL

Before we find a purpose in life, it is important to differentiate between what is important and what is not. Pain helps to select this because it is attached to healing, has no boundaries and is connected to the entire universe. A purpose is attached to something important for you and others.

This mission brings love and joy to the world. How do you recognize a mission? What is a mission? Please take the time to watch carefully. You will find one for you or perhaps you will realize you already have one without being aware of it. A mission helps one to live better and longer. It does not create emptiness around the person but on the contrary it fills up this person's life and spare time. It may be only breathing and being. It may be taking care of our mind and body. It could be not to look for what we want but to enjoy with others what we have. It could be praying for peace in the world. It could be developing dreams for a community, building rainbows, supporting others in this community, becoming a victim advocate, defending human rights, developing long term friendships, being and giving more time to spirituality to make the world a better place, instead of just doing activities. It could be going back to the true self which is to be authentic and spontaneous. It could be many other endless possibilities and horizons, such as to drop the mask covering our personality, to get in touch with the real person we are, and to do something good for others. It could be to care for people in our life, to raise a family and to bring them happiness. It could be to improve our work environment and assist colleagues with difficult tasks. It could be to protect and support the ones we love. It could be to plant flowers, to watch the sun rise and set, to share this beauty and harmony with others. It could be to paint, to write, to play a musical instrument and to create a better environment where to heal our life and other broken hearts.

Sometimes our purpose in life can be found at work. It is possible for teams to work towards a mission and achieve outstanding results. Members are usually selected because they work well together and have synergy. Telepathy is their connector and it gives more power to team members working towards the same goal. These people do not have to discuss issues since they know they will agree on the solutions. They take the same direction without needing to consult and give the best of themselves. Communication is deep at the soul and mind level. Team members write notes on restaurant napkins and have ideas in their dreams. These are often noted on paper in the middle of the night. This approach helps a team to succeed in many difficult situations and can be a purpose in life for one or all of the team members.

It is interesting to note that you are usually alone when you are in pain and you are also alone when you find your mission in life. Trust becomes very important, as does disassociating from people with negative energy who may ultimately try to destroy your dreams. A purpose in life may appear to you at 4:00 a. m. when you wake up to examine your unsatisfied emotional needs. Strangely, the needs of being supported and loved, of receiving respect and recognition, of feeling a personal realization or of belonging to a group without being a burden, might become clear to you in the middle of the night. If we identify our needs, we know ourselves much better, we establish what is important to us and we get clues on what our purpose in life should bring back to us and others. Consequently we select the right track in our life journey. We then decide to stop pretending and achieve our targets.[50]

Once a mission is realized, it must be developed. Intuition is critical in making correct decisions and implementing them. Signs will continue to guide you through hidden areas where your mission will grow. Consequences on others need to be assessed to ensure we will maintain peace and not hurt anyone. Your body will adjust to the needs imposed by your mission. Do you wish to visit people with a car? Your mind will instruct your body to be strong enough to drive. You should envision yourself as healthier and physically capable to achieve your goals in order for you to reach your targets and overcome difficulties.[51] Relationships make understandable the meaning of our mission in life and we achieve when we are open to others. Several components, including the desire not to compete, trust and happiness, decrease pain and bring peace.[52] You can find these resources in yourself. Albert Camus, the French novelist who died at the age of 47 in a car accident, wrote that in the middle of winter, he found in himself an invincible summer.[53] This attitude will lead to success in implementing a mission in life and reaching peace during pain. This is the essential.

CONCLUSION

HEAVEN OF HELL OR HELL FROM HEAVEN

Pain is part of life and regardless of how painful your life is, the earth will not stop turning for you. Pain inhabits Christian life as well as Buddhist life and lives of every other denomination. Some Christians see it as a way to salvation, almost as a source of joy and compassion.[1] In Northern America and Europe suffering is seen as an injustice or failure but in the Orient suffering is less "dramatic" and death is viewed as a passage.[2] This view has value because blame and criticism have a negative impact upon peace of mind, and peace of mind is essential to healing.

> If you keep suffering away from your pain, you find peace and you do not hurt so much.
>
> Dr. Claude M. Roberto.

Some Buddhists view happiness as "a form of suffering" since happiness is fragile and disappears easily. Fortunately religious practices help to transcend this pain found in the body and the mind before reaching *nirvana*.[3] Positive emotions turned to others' well-being bring peace, and real happiness comes from the inside. Imagery, connecting, looking at pain and transforming it into something else such as altruism or compassion, will help to decrease pain.[4]

The first of the Buddhist noble truths is the truth of suffering. This teaching presents pain as normal and is similar to the western and Christian philosophy of seeing pain as a means to becoming a better person. Most religions find meaning in pain and promote the belief that pain is not a waste, but rather brings compassion and strength.[5] The notion that pain improves the sufferer may be distasteful because this idea seems to support suffering as being something good. The key to understanding pain is to distinguish it from suffering. Pain and suffering are not good in themselves. It is what you do when in pain that makes the difference. If you master the maintenance of a steadfast focus away from pain, you may achieve a transcendence unavailable to those who are void of pain. In contrast, if pain becomes a fixation, suffering will result. In fact one can fixate on imaginary pain and some suffering will ultimately result.

Illness can change your life and we often suffer before discovering our priorities in life. It is important to believe pain is never a punishment and we have the power, through the mind and hard work, to

> Truth is what one consciously or unconsciously decides to believe. You are healthy when you don't focus on suffering.
>
> Dr. Claude M. Roberto.

reduce suffering and find peace. This is not always easy because we may see our pain affecting our loved ones and/ or we may live in the wrong environment. In the search for peace, it is important to keep a firm grasp on the mind. Your mind will help focus on your blessings, help eliminate suffering and ultimately find peace. Happiness is not dependent on how you feel but on how your mind reacts to pain and loss.

THE TEACHINGS FROM PAIN

People may not be responsible for the injury, disease or source of their pain although most conditions are known to be connected in some way to beliefs and emotions. People are 100% accountable for their experiences. Even if pain allows transformation, it is not always nec-

> *The mind is its own place and in itself can make a Heaven of Hell, a Hell of Heaven.*
>
> John Milton, cited by Lawrence, Rosch, Plowden, 1998, p. 81.

essary to make us better people in practical life. Even if pain can take people to a higher spirituality, it does not automatically open the gates to paradise. It does not always make us more religious even if it is a constant reminder of the fragility of life and existence of death. Preoccupation with pain is not productive. It causes emotional suffering, costs money, destroys relationships, separates families, causes unemployment, and generally complicates everything. Working outside home, raising a family or maintaining quality of life take on extraordinary challenges. It is not well considered in our western world to perceive pain as a teacher and we see it more as a symptom.[6] This view causes suffering.

Often pain is simply a matter of common sense. Are you short of breath? Maybe you should stop smoking. Pain often tells us it is time to take care of our body.[7] If it causes real tragedies, chronic pain forces to think and find some deeper meaning or purpose in life because a life preoccupied with pain can be viewed as a waste. No one chooses to feel useless, therefore it is essential to define a mission in life in order to focus and give a meaning to a life with pain. The environment around chronic pain tends to become toxic because of the complexity of dealing with pain, because of the suffering attached to it, and because not everyone can transcend it. A change in surroundings with unconditional love and support is one way to grow and feel better.

> Three prerequisites are necessary for deep personal growth: great faith, great doubt, great determination.
>
> Dr. Paul S. Sussman.

A life in pain is never a failure *ipso facto*. Pain teaches us that we have the strength to keep going even after we believe life is impossible. Pain teaches us we can go beyond our limits even if it is not obvious at the time.

Pain can facilitate personal growth, transcendence, understanding, fresh eyes to see the world, compassion, communication, empathy and bidirectional sympathy. If you have an invisible illness (such as chronic pain with no visible physical challenges), don't always expect to receive compassion. Many people will doubt the existence of your pain even if you can show proof of disability. In addition many will treat you as an addict if you use medication to reduce the impact of an invisible illness. In these last two situations, you may have to change your environment to get any beneficial teachings from pain and to allow pain to bring you change and transformation.[8]

Your pain may destroy many relationships. However at the same time, pain may allow new connections in the medical field, in the community, in the family or at work. It can create new links between clients and therapists who seem to benefit and learn from each client. Pain management is a complex professional field, one that is always moving towards the newest approach. Clients also learn a lot from therapists. New connections develop between people in pain. Your therapists may experience pain because it is universal and as clients experiencing pain, you may be able to teach them something. Others can also benefit from painful conditions in a world where pain is a constant evolving field of medical and psychological research.

> People must believe in each other and feel it can be done. Then we are enormously strong. We must keep up each other's courage.
>
> Vincent Van Gogh, painter experiencing chronic pain.

Pain teaches us how to make choices, grow, relax, love ourselves and others, be free with new psychological skills and move from a docile patient's position into active leadership role inspiring others. It allows healing a broken life or heart which we would not have recognized as damaged without the physical pain worsening with emotional suffering when we are in the wrong environment. Pain provides opportunities to volunteer in the field of pain, as a sort of light growing in the dark, working to improve other peoples' lives and to make the world a better place to be in. From a patient's position we can become a model for others and learn to believe in each other to make healing possible.

A serious medical condition teaches that pain exists and may lead us to believe

> And it's primarily the one who is dealing with the disease who does the loving and the healing and the teaching...If you love, you can never be a failure.
>
> Siegel, 2001, p. 249.

that it is incumbent upon ourselves to transform this pain into joy.[9] Pain forces us to take care of ourselves, even if we are very busy juggling a career and parental responsibilities. It shows us that life can be cruel and where to obtain assistance and comfort. Pain teaches us to understand what is essential in life since the essential, in the same way as pain, is invisible to the human eye. It forces us to use our minds and our hearts, and helps to develop stronger relationships and continuous connection with our children because we come to know how fragile and precious life is. Chronic pain allows entry into a timeless extraordinary space where the mind removes the pain or reverts to reversed wellness.[10] After all, healing is a matter of time and opportunity.[11]

Pain teaches us how to recognize synchronicity or providence all day long because we learn to focus attention to signs around us resulting from a need to analyze any opportunity for possible relief. It causes us become more creative because we generally feel better when we create beauty around us and find inspiration in pain rather than fight it at all cost. A close link exists between pain, art and creativity. This could be the result of pushing the body to the extreme, such as done by dancers, music composers or writers who use their bodies and minds to the maximum.

> The worst relation to pain for a dancer or athlete is simply to resist it... The art would lie in discovering how to avoid merely stiff, passive resistance and how to use the pain as the medium for a fluid, creative performance, even if the performance were limited to walking downstairs for dinner or climbing behind the wheel of a car.
>
> Morris cited by Dillard, 2002, p. 391.

Pain teaches us to feel better by sharing time, money and energy. Generosity allows connecting with others which is so essential for well-being and forces us to ultimately find our level of resilience. It allows us to seek and find a purpose to pursue in life. This goal is the keystone which prevents pain from defeating us and allows us to transcend its effects. Opening our hearts to unconditional love can become a purpose in life beginning with ourselves and extending to others. Since much money is not required, when we decide "to give from the heart", generosity should be affordable to all. Pain starting in the body before extending to the mind then becomes a universal matter where much remains to be discovered.

DEC, 3, 2007
FEB. 11, 2011

WHAT IS HEALING?

The root word of healing, "to hale," means "to make whole,"[12] "to be in harmony." Thus healing does not involve returning to the physical, psychological and spiritual state in which we existed prior to the onset of the disease, illness or injury. The definition for the word is very subjective; basically it means what you want it to mean and what makes you feel good.

> There is no reality, and it wouldn't matter if there were. All that exists are various points of view. There are no rules.
>
> Dr. Paul S. Sussman

Harmony

Harmony establishes a balance with an altered situation, and healing occurs at the physical, psychological and spiritual levels. It is a complex process involving the client and a healer or group of caregivers. It combines knowledge from different therapists inviting the client in pain into a relationship.[13] Healing is then "a dialogue and a learning experience" for the client and the therapist.[14] The final result is an increase in inner strength, knowledge and enlightenment. Real healing goes beyond therapy, and increases abilities. The power acquired from healing increases the ability to tolerate pain.

Hippocrates, a 5th century B. C. Greek physician, believed pain came from a change in physical condition resulting from excess, deprivation or contrasts in temperature, and healing was a return to harmony. Medications, and other forces, helped to heal and make another change at this time to improve physical condition.[15] During this era, Plato, an ancient Greek philosopher, developed the premise that thoughts, originating from intelligence, are reflected on the body, especially the liver. If these thoughts are threatening, contractions and pain occur and if they are peaceful, relaxation occurs and freedom is brought to the organs.[16]

Magic

The Greek philosopher, Socrates, who lived from 469 to 399 B.C., is known to us through writings by Plato. Socrates' approach to healing led him to search what to be the proper conduct in life. He explained that an effective agent to remove headache pain needed a magical formula added to a plant component. He believed the entire body should be treated. In the case of physical illness, he suggested the soul, where the good and the bad originate, as well as the entire body, needed care. This magical formula was said to cure the soul. An example of such a formula was a speech with positive or wise thoughts being able to bring health to the body. These words were believed to keep the head and the entire body in healthy condition.

Whole knowledge

According to Socrates, many physicians made the mistake of being specialists of the soul or the body without combining treatments to both. He insisted that the soul needed to be cured before the body, even if both required care to heal.[17] In his view healing signified improved mental and moral well-being and one would not occur without the other. The first responsibility of physicians was said to have been to know their own souls because the soul was the basis for the person. A thorough knowledge of the various body parts was simply to know what was personally owned and not who owned it. Consequently physicians who knew only anatomy and not themselves should not have been in charge of curing people. Healers conduct valuable activities only when they touch other people's souls.[18]

Beauty

Florence Nightingale believed every woman was a nurse.[19] She cared for approximately 4,000 patients during the Crimean Wars (1854-1856) although experiencing herself chronic pain. Her publications became the foundation for universal health care. In July 1865 she wrote she was "even more broken in mind than in body" and suffered from "such horrible loneliness,"[20] which added to her physical pain. Her illness provided her the time to write for the benefit of mankind. She mentioned that many books had been written "upon the effect of mind upon the body", agreeing that this impact was real. At the same time she wished for "a little more was thought of the effect of the body on the mind."[21] She believed healing came from a number of other sources, including direct sunlight influencing "upon the spirits" and "upon the human body."[22]

Other sources of beauty including colors, forms, objects, landscapes, flowers, growing plants, pets and children were also components essential for recovery. She remembered "a nosegay of wild flowers sent to me, and from that moment recovery becoming more rapid."[23] Beauty, and sunlight, were therapy for recovery of "health and spirit."[24] She recommended that hospitals be constructed with large low windows to allow the ill to see landscapes from their beds.

Freedom

Healing is removing suffering from the mind and enabling energy to be free to concentrate on new dreams. It is a victory increasing quality of life and allowing the mind to be at peace. Healing is writing our own life guidelines based on personal experiences and not hearsay.

> The sun is not only a painter but a sculptor...Put the pale withering plant and human being into the sun, and, if not too far gone, each will recover health and spirit.
>
> About care to the sick, Nightingale, 1946, p. 48 – 49.

Transformation

Healing involves deep transformation, otherwise defense system, including pain and tension, remains, otherwise physical and mental conditions stay unchanged; recovery is then impossible.

Retreat

In Buddhism and Shamanism healing is part of the process of lucidity, awareness (where healing begins and suffering starts to cease) and mindfulness (which is a practice of meditation). Meditation space can be just like a hospital where our regular activities cease and we retreat into solitude awaiting a cure. Meditation allows the mind, body and world to be one and to reach healing.[25] A special area in the home or the garden can be reserved to enjoy silence. Unfortunately our modern lives are filled with too much noise, even in public areas with cell phones and radios, and silence is necessary to heal. Quiet time allows us to maintain an inner life. Silence may of course bring back inner issues and wounds because nothing distracts us, but it is necessary to know them in order to find solutions and to heal.

> **Wellness demands a transformation at the core of the intellect. Paradoxically, it is illness which often presents us with a wonderful opportunity to achieve this transformation.**
> Greenwood and Nunn, 1994, p. 96.

Awareness

Healing is recognizing good health forces and synchronicity that will reduce your pain. It is paying attention to the world around us when making decisions that can change our life because these decisions may also impact others. Only the decisions with a positive impact should be implemented because a negative impact on you or others will of course not bring healing. You can't heal independently from others. In the journey for peace with pain, a few significant moments will serve as crossroads and your intuition will help you to see the signs and to find the right path leading you to healing.

Self care

Healing is loving and listening to yourself, offering you kindness and taking care of yourself, not only physically but also mentally and spiritually. It will ask you to choose physicians, healers, allied health specialists (psychologists, nurses, chiropractors, physical and massage therapists), priests and caregivers. They will teach you how to manage your perception of pain and develop improved abilities to accomplish it. Caring for yourself also includes paying attention to small things, which may serve as alerts for further medical investigation. When continual pain is a daily companion, we tend to focus on it and disregard other potential illness, such as cancer or cardio-vascular related disease. Intractable pain requires a large supply of energy and can hide unrelated medical symptoms. Your commitment should be to your entire body and recognize signs of potential hazards to your health. This is essential as pain can predispose our bodies to further illness.

Acceptance

Healing is asking society to accept us, even if we are different than what we were before. It is accepting the changes (resulting from injury, disease or illness) that forced our bodies to age in a short period of time, our finances to decrease, our relationships to change. They may cause our work and marriage to sometimes disappear or be disrupted, our past activities and priorities to change and our beliefs to be updated. This potentially painful shift will likely be one of the most significant challenges we will be forced to undertake. Our previous world with friends and family may undergo catastrophic disintegration and we may become unsure as to what our upcoming years will bring. Friends and families may not feel the change the way we do because their priorities, activities and belief systems can remain the same. We are the ones who will need develop a different lifestyle and systems to facilitate healing.

Sharing

Healing is considering that we are a part of the same universe, open to world issues and caring for others. One major and very common mistake is to believe men must be separated one from the other and be also different in order to succeed. On the contrary, people are connected. They live together in communities, parishes, or neighborhoods if they want to be healthy. Since pain is universal and since devastations are continually spread by the media, healing requires being aware of global suffering and tragedy. Healing is as personal, when dealing with body injuries, as it is universal, when facing a tsunami disaster such as the one in Southern Asia in 2004. Sharing often includes crying for ourselves and for others. Tears do not need words to express thoughts and they are an excellent way to offer a message of pain and support. This type of communication is even an honor we reserve for only a few people because it is such a personal occurrence.

> Only a day lived for others is a life worthwhile day.
>
> Albert Einstein

Communications

Healing, just like a flu epidemic, is communicable. This means it allows the development of ties based on love and friendship, and it gives us the opportunity to rediscover together small pleasures in nature, such as a sunset or a visit to a garden.

Healing is developing open communications with physicians assisting us in ways that may be outside their formal training. It is exchanging ideas with other people to give them hope and encouragement. It is also forcing caregivers to communicate internally.

The causes of chronic pain are manifold and treatment often involves a number of highly trained experts. Specialists report findings to family physicians and in Alberta have recently begun entering their findings into a central data base accessible only by medical professionals. Despite these advances communication between physicians and consumers can be a continuing challenge. "Discrepancies between what the doctor sees and what the patient feels occur in most diseases, because sickness is not caused by disease, but by disturbed function, and function involves a complex set of phenomena with physiological, psychological and cultural dimensions."[26] Healing relates to all of these components and forces us to communicate with others.

Melting fear

Healing is breathing which gives life, brings oxygen to the brain, removes toxins, clears thoughts and promotes positive physiological and psychological changes. Healing removes fear even if the causes of pain are not managed and consequences are unknown. One of the worst pains can be the result of fear of loss of life, independence, income, spouse, relationships, and significant friends.[27] Pain is a complex issue with physiological origins, pain extends to work, finances, social life and intimacy with others. If you are struggling with a toxic workplace, marriage, family or friends, fear is unavoidable. Fear can cause additional stress and physical pain. If you live with fear, healing is likely impossible. Healing demands that you release fear.

> All healing is essentially the release of all fear.
> Dr. Paul S. Sussman from anonymous source.

Simple image

It can be said that a healer or a caregiver does not really heal but holds a mirror. Here the therapist guides the client in pain to see himself/herself and presents an image of what the client

> **Fear is a very powerful weapon...Don't act out of fear.**
> From *The Sea Inside*, a 2004 Spanish movie by Alejandro Amenábar.

could become. It is the client's role to decide whether he/she chooses to select the image.[28] Healing can be also simply establishing or re-establishing balance and harmony, sometimes only with relationships or placebos, or with the mirror held by the therapist. The balance is achieved between the physical, emotional, intellectual and spiritual dimensions.[29] However the right environment and support are usually necessary for the person in pain to reach this image or balance. If they are not available, the client in pain has to develop them, if needed with help from the therapist.

Relationship

The Greek physician Hippocrates wrote: "Some patients, though conscious that their condition is perilous, recover their health simply through their contentment with the goodness of the physician."[30] A positive response removing pain and other symptoms (such as fear or muscle spasms) created with the assistance of physical and/or psychological interventions, is much more attainable if care is provided by a compassionate physician. To re-establish harmony, the therapeutic alliance is essential. Medication is a common pain reduction method. However some caring physicians have the power to alleviate fear and improve the client's comfort irrespective of medication. In my experience the therapeutic relationship is a most important factor in healing; one that generally is neglected. The client-doctor relationship is truly the first pillar of healing.[31] In my experience the quality of the healing relationship (rather than the technique) is the hidden foundation of healing. The bond between physician and client results from compassion, trust, empathy, and a mutual willingness to move forward. The healer and the client can be one in their pain because in the process of care for one another, this unity or wholeness heals both parties. Certainly we heal together and no one should ever leave a doctor's office without hope. Everyone holds healing potential[32] and meditation may help to develop this potential. Communication and a bond between the client and therapist must be deep enough to transform pain into something more acceptable and to allow the client to be at peace with pain.

Healing may also involve agreeing to follow advice from health specialists whose practice is flawed due to defense procedures they use to protect themselves from discipline and litigation. Many professionals work under strict rules and policies of professional associations and other governing bodies, and care for you even if it is not permissible for them to make this evident. They may also need healing. It is your responsibility to add them to your team and develop a therapeutic alliance with those who care the most for you and provide the most effective treatment.

> Medicine is not only a science but also the art of letting our own individuality interact with the individuality of the patient.
>
> Schweitzer in Carlson and Shield, 1989, p. 83.

Healing is of course interacting with others able to provide hope and support removing isolation and despair.

Healing facilitates wholeness. Pain often creates feelings of abandonment. Empathic bonding with the medical team and significant others makes us stronger because it allows hope and sharing, both leading to peace.

Peace

Healing can be a peaceful preparation for death. Healing is not reserved for the sick. It is good for all mankind and forces us to become more inclusive, more capable of loving and developing relationships. In a sense, it remains a sort of mystery.[33]

Plan

Healing is following a recovery plan that may include several methods of dealing with pain. Various traditional and non traditional approaches are explained in this book. Consumers face choices with activities and treatments they wish to follow.

> *Healing, wherever and however it occurs, brings each person and humanity as a whole toward a more inclusive, more unobstructed relatedness to all that is emerging in this adventure of life.*
>
> Moss in Carlson and Shield, 1989, p. 37.

Conventional medicine is based on a scientific approach whereas alternative therapies are developed from the concept that illness results from a blockage of energy and lack of balance and harmony.

Healing is selecting a medical approach or integration of different systems of medicine. We have included four models in this book. The first one, allopathic or western medicine, includes passive patients, and is often very limited in its capacity for dealing with people living with chronic pain. Scientific medicine involves licensed physicians, support staff, the use of technology, medication and related therapies. This is a biomedical approach with formal relationships between physicians and clients. Unfortunately in my experience it does not work optimally for chronic pain.

Western medicine is also limited because technology rarely allows clear and measurable proof of pain. It establishes relationships with physicians trained to interpret objective X rays and laboratory test results. However, it is not well designed to deal with invisible and highly subjective experiences that are modified by variables such as the resistance and relaxation practices.

Healing is visiting these physicians and developing a therapeutic alliance even though the intensity of pain is not apparent from most medical or laboratory tests. The western approach provides access to medication very often required for pain management. This western system is dominant in Northern America and Europe, and has the most extensive insurance coverage.

Behavioral medicine includes physicians and allied health specialists such as nurses, psychologists, chiropractors, and massage therapists. It is a relatively new approach that encourages the one in pain to remain active through exercise, nutritional food, and psychological and relaxation practices. This second medical system is an approach that often works well for people with chronic pain.

The third system, transcendental medicine, is also fairly new in our society but has existed for at least 20, 000 years in other cultures. This approach does not involve organized professionals. The client in pain follows guidelines from healers, clergy, family and community, and can be active or passive. The word "transcendental" means "beyond self" and the healer often goes into a trance or altered state of consciousness with the person experiencing pain. This system assumes an invisible force connects people and comes from God or a healing force. It involves touch, prayers, sacred places, ceremonies and tools to alter consciousness, with the goal to find balance and harmony. Chinese medicine, the fourth system, embraces acupuncture and other practices based on the flow of energy in the body and is followed by many people around the world.

Healing is the willingness to try these systems[34] with a positive attitude and later defining the best components for individual situations. It is fighting for good quality time with physicians. It is agreeing to laboratory tests and invasive procedures that stand at the base of our traditional Northern American system of care. This system has been slow to recognize chronic pain as an illness and is able to define it only by ruling out other medical conditions. Healing is willing to be also integrative in accepting spirituality and mystical links with the universe as well as a supreme force. It is reaching beyond the illness and considering it as a confirmation of the need to heal. It becomes even more complex when the medical issue disappears and pain remains as in the case of phantom pain. Healing is connected to the body, mind and spirit, as well as cultural traditions and involves the one in pain as an active participant at the same level as families, communities and health specialists.

Healing is recovery even if the causes of pain are unknown, highly subjective and cultural.[35] Therefore it is often advisable to focus on recovery if causes are not essential to healing. We recommend integrative medicine including both conventional and alternative therapies. You should select the therapies or approaches you believe to be compatible and to work best for you. There is not a miracle solution and you may need to investigate several therapies before defining which ones you prefer and consequently, defining at the same time your own healing.

Interpretation

Healing is knowing how to prevent, revert or accept pain and, although pain is experienced by several millions people, healing is personal and needs to be discovered by each individual. Healing results from the meaning we give to chronic pain, from its purpose in life, from the belief of self-value and from the power of imagination. A healer is someone who supports clients learning to trust their own inner truths and their intuition while learning to live more fully and freely.[36]

Passion

Healing means passion attached to creativity, to love and interdependence among living and non-living things such as family and nature. Passion allows us to introduce beauty in our lives with gardens, flowers, music, songs, painting, writing and other forms of art. Beauty helps to keep us healthy; relaxes and distracts; it seems to attract peace and happiness because it connects with perfection and the invisible. Passion helps to find beauty because if we love something or someone, we make it beautiful and essential. We then forget our pain.

> I see creativity as an ocean, a flow, the water we swim in. It is the source of the waves that heal.
>
> Conrad-Da'oud, in Carlson and Shield, 1989, p. 98.

Love

Love for the person to be healed and for the healer is the common denominator connecting the many forms of healing. Love is synonymous with care; it is important here because it is the most significant element in human life. If the therapist does not care for the client, healing will not take place. If the client does not care enough for himself or herself and for the therapist, healing suggestions from the therapist will not be followed. To maintain integrity and trust therapists must live the suggested healing message they send to clients. They must show them they are lovable in order for healing to take place. Of course the healing suggested message helping clients to feel better can be different for each healer. This message is important because it is the magical formula healing the ones with pain. It may be modified according to clients' needs. People with pain often connect with a therapist presenting what they believe to be the most relevant message to them. The healing process is a dialogue and a learning experience for client and therapist, and benefits both because healers often look at their own pain and emotions when they deal with their clients' pain.[37] Love between the healer and the client helps to restore the energy flow of the body and in addition to be a love between two persons, it is also love for harmony and peace allowing healing.[38]

Finding the essential

Healing is personal development because it includes intimate decisions and hard work. Effective therapy gives the one experiencing pain "a clear vision of what he or she needs to do as well as the strength and integration of mind, body and spirit to do it."[39] You will need to decide if you will remove the causes and triggers from your life identified as the sources or aggravating factors. In order to change a toxic environment or update surroundings not matching your new priorities and your need to heal, you may decide to seek out a new job and new relationships.

You then implement your decisions before healing commences. When the struggle becomes too difficult, many therapies are available to guide you in this book. Those seeking healing must learn how to focus and identify the essentials before implementing what is the most important. Healing is then living your life just as if you will die tonight. So pick the essentials and do what really matters to you. You will feel better.[40]

Education

The therapist empowers – and not overpowers – the clients by stimulating their own energy and educating them about their own resources.[41] This personal growth involves removing obstructions to our natural state in order to re-establish harmony and wholeness in our lives.[42] Well-being is possible only if we remove the dark shadows of our life which are issues buried very deeply in our psyche to be solved in order to heal. These hidden patches of shade cause additional pain, poison our happiness and prevent medication from reducing pain. We should all deal with them in order to become free and feel better. The healer empowers us to look within for healing and disease is a message telling us we have deviated from our true path.[43] Hippocrates was the first in the 5th century B.C. to write that the natural healing force, within each one of us, is the greatest force in getting well.[44]

Decision

Healing is being in harmony within ourselves and its existence between ourselves and others. This requires establishing priorities according to the impact they have on your health. It is rejecting "black holes" or negative people depressing your physical, mental and spiritual levels, and it is introducing new people and new components into your life in order to facilitate healing. It is deciding to enjoy life and selecting who will be your companions in the quest for peace. Healing is not feeling guilty about the impact of our health issues on friends, family and work. Healing is also about believing we have value and bring something to the world.

Compassion

It has been said that illness is an opportunity to healing even if pain is not beneficial. Illness forces us to assess where we are going and what is the most important to us. It pushes us to evaluate how we care for ourselves.[45] Healing is about being compassionate for us and for others. It is looking at the present and building for the future. It is about extending our field of actions and making them a benefit to us and others. Then it allows you to develop a mission in life, spread joy around you, paint a rainbow which allows altruism and realization of something beautiful for everyone. This new goal will force you to choose your most essential battles and your own causes which will bring something good to the world. It means persevering through pain to realize the dream and integrating pain into our lives instead of resisting it. If you fight against pain, so capricious and impossible to control, your energy will be depleted in this battle instead of offering a contribution to our universe. Sometimes healing does not include a physical improvement in the level of pain. Release of pain, then, can come from the determination to perform a compassionate and loving act for others.[46]

> Of course they needed to care. It was the meaning of everything.
> Lowry, 1993, p. 157.

Trust

Healing is trusting in life and the strength of human nature even if physicians and others tell you your pain will be there for ever, even if your friends and family don't believe in your recovery. Healing is about having a sacred place to rest, meditate, breathe and listen in silence. This place could be a garden, inside your mind or around the house, or could be a quiet room in your home. You enter this place each time when you want to feel better. This place that you trust, is a shelter always available to you.

Perseverance

Healing is rehabilitation with happiness. It is also crying because tears release negative emotions and losses lodged in us. Healing is letting these destructive seeds go away so that they do not grow and make us dependent on them. It is getting up in the morning with a smile and dreaming in our mind even if our body hurts and even if we are lonely. Healing is accepting what hurts and can't be changed; it is also reducing the importance of this negative component in our life. It is ongoing work on what is important, positive and connected to our dreams.

Giving

Healing is giving of yourself. Relationships, which tie you to others, allow you to feel better not because of what you receive but because of what you give. Some of

> **When your heart is in your dreams, your dreams come true.**
>
> Walt Disney, filmmaker, from movie Pinocchio

us will remember these recommendations so beautifully expressed by St. Francis of Assisi, the Italian medieval poet born in 1182 in Umbria: "Grant that I may not so much seek to be consoled as to console; to be understood as to understand; to be loved as to love; for it is in giving that we receive." Most Christians and others have heard these touching words, but people usually ignore that St. Francis suffered from intense chronic pain caused by a degenerative disease of the lungs, stomach and bones. Giving himself and connecting with nature were his way of healing.

Nature and spirituality

The theory stating human beings are made of earth and water is present in several mythologies such as Pandora in the Greek myth and Eve in the Hebrew myth. Mud has been a healing agent for millennia, and is still therapy today for joints and skin, as well as relaxation. On the scientific level, human life biologically develops with water in a fluid environment; air and water are indispensable throughout this life. Mud contains magnesium, potassium, calcium, chromium, silica, and other minerals. Cleopatra treasured it and Pliny, a Roman writer, explained its therapeutic quality. St. John reported that Jesus anointed a blind beggar's eyes with mud to return his sight.[47] St. Francis of Assisi, in the *Canticle of the Sun* (approximately 1224 AD) called the sun, air and fire his brothers, and the earth, moon, stars and water his sisters. This notion of brotherhood and sisterhood with the universe is parallel with the components associated with the *chakras*. Fire is also essential and in Greek mythology we owe fire to Prometheus, who stole it

> And regarding the ones enduring disabiliting illnesses and pain, may they be happy, these ones who endure in peace, they will be crowned by You, the Highest.
>
> St. Francis of Assisi, 1182 – 1226, *Canticle of the Sun*, translation from Italian by the authors.

from Zeus and brought it to earth. St. Francis wrote his piece of poetry at the end of his life, experiencing intense physical pain. It is then not surprising he ended his *Canticle of the Sun* by stating the need for the disabled and the ill to maintain peace in what we believe to be nature.

In Asian beliefs, forces from the *chakras* connecting us with peace, nature and with other human beings bring healing. As a consequence, walks along rivers, sea shores, in woods, gardening and any peaceful activities that put us in close touch with nature are healing. Connecting with others and being interdependent should also ensure this peaceful link with nature.

Healing is difficult to define and each of us can use different words, based on differing beliefs, to express a same state of interior peace. We believe healing comes from missions helping others, from collectivity and from ordinary activities found in extraordinary relationships. Of course these pursuits include a component of beauty and a link with nature; they also require unconditional love as well as compassion. Healing is also letting go of worries and keeping them at a distance so that they don't hurt us. Healing generates from powerful positive forces that come from nature and various sources depending on the believers' background. They can be a divinity, God or the four elements found in the seven *chakras*: earth, water, air, fire, or unconditional love located in the heart, or cosmic energy. These forces fight illnesses and prevent their development. Faith is more important than the exact definition of the forces.

Vision

Healing techniques might be followed in order to reach recovery and your job is to select the best ones suited to you. Therapists should not get bagged down in their favored techniques because the client is then almost regarded as a subject for the practice. Each person has unique needs and may require different techniques. The therapists' care and unconditional love are more important than the techniques, and they can be transferred through these techniques. This process of transfer is important.[48] The person seeking healing, and the bond formed with the therapist impact the success of the techniques. Healing comes from the brain and the heart, from a place deep in the body. Happiness and well-being do not exist on the periphery. Healing is meant to be as complex as pain and to fill up our interior emptiness. Trees have beautiful leaves, rose bushes have exquisite scents and gorgeous flowers, and they survive winter because of life held deeply within their roots, and so do we as human beings.

Everyone does well to develop a personal recipe or vision for healing and each process should involve medication, compassion and altruism because of the human interconnectedness of all beings. We hope you will find your mission in life, realize a dream and reach your own form of healing.

THE ART OF HAPPINESS

Health does not automatically lead to happiness however happiness is essential to health. A commitment to many things is needed to be happy. You need to agree to live in the present and enjoy it, and one of the requirements then is to stop the race with time. Happiness is a choice and you face this dilemma: Do I continue to race against time by increasing the number of things in my life or do I decide to increase the amount of life I put into the things I select-ed to do?[49] Only then you look for your priorities, also known as your mission, and ensure you devote to them sufficient time and energy. For example, if your children are a priority, you commit to them a large part of your time, many other things will wait. This should not bother or annoy you as long as you are able to identify and follow your priorities.

> I decided to be happy because it is good for my health.
>
> Voltaire, French philosopher and writer, cited by André, 2003, p. 10.

Another very important activity is responsibility for your health. You pursue your healing. This is anoth-er priority you should not abandon to others. You are an important piece in the large puzzle holding the world together and you would do well to not neglect this link in the chain.

A part of this therapy you provide to yourself, is to decide to enjoy life with the people you love and to believe it is possible to connect with these people even at a dis-tance. In our modern world, distance and number of times you spent with the ones you love, can be an issue making happiness more difficult. So, please don't forget that inten-sity of feelings in your relationships is more significant than distance and number of hours spent with loved ones. Consider life as a bank account or, if you prefer, a trea-sure box. Fill the box with little pleasures and review them when you experience a trying time. What could you col-lect in your little box? Let's see... why not photos of your family at different dates and times, images of your garden, music notes, a drawing or a sentence meaning something very special? When you need comfort, open the box and play with its content until you feel better. In reality this does not require a physical box and you could very well hold your little treasures within yourself. Your mind will be there to open the box for you during times of need.

Happiness is an art because it is the result of a creation involving natural skills and hard work. It is a victory over suffering. Because happiness is a representation, it can be learned at some future date after the time of victory over pain, when your mind can recall happy moments of the past to reduce suffering.[50] Yes, happiness is not automatically given to anyone but can be created. Social success does not always bring happiness, and fairy tales are wrong when they say people get married and live happily ever after. Healing, happiness and well-being are never acquired for ever. All three result from resilience, hard work, artistic creation, renewed actions, ongoing attitudes and solid connections with significant people in our lives.

Well-being is not happiness, it is feeling good in the present and it remains largely a perception. Happiness is a representation of well-being because of good memories or anticipation of good upcoming feelings.[51]

Strangely enough, even if happiness has a positive impact on our health, happiness is not always well received. Most everyone is more attracted by stories of disaster rather than tales of happiness. In our world, as soon as you watch cartoons, or pick up the paper or turn on your TV or radio, you are bombarded with reports on war, violence and destruction. These media reports tend to attract interest and sell newspapers

> *Pain is reduced through the right connections with the right people and these relationships are extremely important in therapy. Otherwise how do you explain that medication provides better results if you get along with your physician?*
>
> Dr. Claude M. Roberto.

and magazines at an ever-increasing rate. Ironically everyone wants to be happy but very few people are comfortable discussing it. This is normal because happiness, as is pain, is difficult to define, identify and understand. It is linked to our private lives, inner values and the meaning we give to life. Many people do not feel comfortable discussing such intimate matters.

The many definitions of happiness

Attempting to define happiness or pleasure is very difficult and challenging because the body, mind and soul are connected. Consequently, happiness is a complex physical, emotional and spiritual experience. It is based on the fulfillment of physical needs and self esteem, and it also has a social dimension since care to others can bring happiness.[52] It is difficult to feel happy without sharing a part of our happiness with others needing happiness in their lives.

We agree it is possible to approach happiness with four verbs: to be, to have, to do, to belong. The first verb describes the act of being happy by just being alive. The second is about the act of owning things we value and feel we require in order to fulfill our needs. The third verb speaks to the necessity of creating and producing works which bring pleasure, and the last verb has to do with connecting with a welcoming family or community.[53]

People in our western culture and Asia have tried for at least the past 2 500 years

> Keep your eyes on that last day, on your dying. Happiness and peace, they were not yours unless at death you can look back on your life and say: I lived, I did not suffer.
>
> Sophocles, *Oedipus the King*, Chorus, 1984 – 1987.

to define happiness, and yet no single definition has been found. Epicurus, the ancient Greek philosopher (born in the 4th century B.C.), considered friends, freedom, food, accommodation, clothes and thought as being a requisite for happiness.[54] For the ancient Greeks, it was necessary to find personal good and public good together, however no one could pretend to be happy throughout a lifetime. Solon, the Greek statesman and poet from the 7th century B.C., even believed no one could claim to be happy before the arrival of death,[55] meaning that happiness could not be identified during life.

Approximately 2 500 B.C., Buddha proposed that cessation of suffering can be caused through the cultivation of non-attachment to the self. He described the path leading to this goal in terms of definitive attitudes, perspectives, day-to-day behaviors and spiritual practices. His followers believe that he attained this goal.

The Greek philosopher Aristotle (4th century B.C.) wrote happiness was the "summum bonum" or "highest good."[56] However happiness, the synonym of harmony and balance for the ancient Greeks, was fragile because of the difficulty in maintaining balance. Aristotle[57] also wrote that happiness is different from all other acquisitions because we search for it and for nothing else. It is the final target. According to Seneca, the Roman writer and philosopher, pain hurts but it is not a bad condition. It can even be positive. It transforms and it is not seen as leading to depression and additional pain if it is controlled and if we know how to be free from pain.[58] This would ensure a good and happy life.

In a sense, happiness is like faith. Some people believe in happiness while others don't, and such is the case with faith. Searching for happiness can divide people because the meaning of the word can be very personal. True happiness comes from the inside. Any type of happiness holds the illusion of being eternal, the hope to last forever and the promise it will be maintained for a long time.[59] People who help others by giving and receiving love are often considered as very happy.

Some forms of pleasure, such as pleasure from revenge, are not happiness and are a hidden form of suffering. Physical health and material security can lead to happiness, but this is not necessarily the case. In addition, painful memories fade more rapidly than happy ones. Thus the perception of happiness is often retrospective and nostalgic. Happiness goes beyond physical fortune because the unhealthy as well as the ill can be happy. Happiness is different from pleasure and goes beyond our physical or psychological limits.[60] When happiness is attained, the ill do not need to pursue healing further, because happiness transcends physical pain. In addition, happiness takes you away from a broken life and heals your heart.

Does pain allow happiness?

Our answer is an affirmative yes! This can occur if certain conditions outlined in this book are met, if you perceive pain as a problem, and not an unjust drama, if you get rid of suffering and reach peace by making the right choices. How do you wish to live your life? Your actions for personal development should help take you away from loneliness and create your own happiness. We cannot provide a magic formula. Happiness remains a mystery born from peace when you connect and when pain is transformed into hope and serenity.

Hope is a powerful ally for the ill seeking happiness. Happiness can be hidden but when the circumstances are favorable, it becomes real even to the ill. In the *Divine Comedy*, a masterpiece of Italian literature, Dante visits hell where he sees the worst a man can see. He visits Lucifer, the emperor of the land of pain. Fortunately he manages, with his friend Virgil, to take a secret path and return fto say: *"E quindi uscimmo a riveder le stelle"* or "And then we came out to see again the stars."[61] If Dante, exiled in real life from his loved city of Florence, returned to enjoy the stars, why would you not recover from pain to enjoy your stars?

What is happiness for people in constant pain?

Like pain, happiness is very complex and subjective. It is better to experience pain and be happy than painless and unhappy. Happiness is also highly subjective because individuals perceive the world in different ways. Some need happiness both at home and work to feel happy, others are comfortable with happiness only at home or work. For many, pleasure from working and productivity[62] increases happiness. Transformation from pain can also lead to peace and happiness.

Sources of pleasure, just as those of pain, are endless and can be found in many activities. These include writing, dancing, producing or listening to music, painting, singing, enjoying nature, decorating, gardening, sewing, practicing sports, raising a family, developing intimacy with the right companion, or entering a sacred place through mental exercise. The seeds of happiness are numerous, however they include the same key components of creativity, connection, energy, awareness and relaxation. People experiencing chronic pain need to make a choice by deciding to avoid suffering and look for sources of pleasure that facilitate enjoyment. Even if total happiness seems to be out of grasp, grabbing crumbs is often possible. Your mind has the ability to transform them into great moments. Unfortunately pessimism often prevents us from gathering them and counting our blessings. Please don't forget to work towards creating your own happiness. Peace and happiness do not appear on their own. Just as pain, happiness is communicable. It is your responsibility to choose and develop instances of joy if you wish to create your own happiness.

Paying attention to nature may be rewarding. Classical philosophers believed that being close to nature was a source of happiness and for most people, paradise can be found in a garden or a peaceful territory.[63] These moments take on a larger dimension if they are shared with others.

Connecting with significant others also removes loneliness and promotes peace and healing. If someone is happy to see you, this person is significant in your life[64] and should be included in your search for happiness. If someone is never mad at you, holds your hand and gives you unconditional support, this person will bring you peace. If you feel comfortable calling someone at 1:00 A.M., you should consider this person as someone important for your healing.

Laughing is a well accepted pain therapy. Connected to happiness, laughing distracts the attention from painful feelings, decreases muscle tension, multiplies endorphins and cultivates optimism.[65] Is laughing the only expression of happiness? Of course not, because otherwise you would be able to obtain happiness from techni-

> When you can't escape and you constantly rely on everyone else, you learn to cry by smiling.
>
> From *The Sea Inside*, a 2004 Spanish movie by Alejandro Amenábar.

cal means. Laughing is not always a sign of happiness even if it is usually attached to happiness.

Senses are our allies in the quest for peace and happiness. They bring us pain, pleasure and therapeutic methods to deal with pain. Many people with chronic pain experience tinnitus or ringing in the ears making relaxation very difficult, if not impossible. On the other end, hearing allows music which decreases negative thoughts and feelings, and muscle tension, and increases endorphin levels to reduce pain.[66] Happiness is possible if the ones in pain teach themselves to engage the senses in finding pleasure rather than disengaging them and suffering.

Finding a meaning to life is not sufficient to be totally happy, but not finding any meaning in life prevents happiness.[67] A life mission helps to focus energy into something good and sail without capsizing. The body will follow your desire to achieve your mission that will remove suffering. Pain without suffering does not hurt as much. So, find a quiet place, do some deep breathing and ask yourself: What is my mission in life? What do I create for others and what benefits do I derive from it? Then, develop strategies and implement them while moving toward your mission in life. The end results need not be extraordinary and will never be finished. For us the essential is to conduct ordinary activities in outstanding relationships.

To be or do are not sufficient for happiness because pleasure asks us to note the effects of these sources on our body, mind and soul. For example, the essential is not to be in the middle of nature but to be aware of cool water, light wind, scents and season colors.[68] Being physically connected to nature is not important because imagination can produce the same awareness. Finally, having a certain amount of freedom, without being alone, and being able to laugh, also play an important role in the search for pleasure and pain relief.[69]

Optimism for the ones in pain

Optimism is essential to grow, be happy, realize something from pain and find peace. In the recent movie by Roberto Benigni, *La Vita è bella* or *Life is beautiful* (1999), a little Jewish boy survives a concentration camp because his father taught him that life is a huge game where it is important to win. Happiness depends largely on removing obstacles. Optimistic attitudes surrounding our skills, trust in ourselves and others are essential. Trust can be difficult for those in pain, and happiness (as we know) is hard work. No one ever said that happiness would be easy to achieve.

An optimist sees hope everywhere, rejects preoccupation with fear and unhappy moments to concentrate instead on joyful experiences, learns from mistakes, does not feel guilty for being happy or feeling well, knows how to relax, trusts others and celebrates minutes when pain decreases. An optimist doesn't foretell future disasters, lives each moment at the time and doesn't review the same issues. An optimist decides in advance to be happy and knows how to create happiness. An optimist retrieves happy moments hidden in memory, loves other people, and feels at ease between medical appointments. Being an optimist is not easy, and being at peace with pain is a reward granted primarily to the optimistic.

> **Being happy is not necessarily being joyful, it is being fully present in what we live.**
>
> D'Ansembourg, 2004, p. 261 translated from French by the authors.

Extraordinary life in an extraordinary space

In conclusion, what is happiness for those in pain? It is being at peace with pain by following the therapies discussed in this book. You should select those suited to your personality and conditions. Being at peace is a deal you agree to with pain for the length of time you follow the therapies you prefer. This means not to seeing pain as unjust or as a disability. It does not mean you will be pain-free but rather it means you will avoid suffering and will be at peace with pain.

What can bring the moments of joy necessary to be at peace and happy? Which ordinary activities in an extraordinary space could you undertake to connect and live without suffering? Opportunities are numerous and these are only examples: Relaxing in a garden, a room or any other sacred space to find a refuge, living with our individual values in a free world, staying in the present and enjoying it without being worried about the past or future, seeing one day at a time on a line rather than compressed in a hard dark ball in front of you, helping others, taking the time to stop, breathe and think before following the "to be, to have, to do and to own" models, being optimistic and appreciating life, developing skills to be happy, doing the maximum each day in order not to be sorry about missed opportunities, building activities bringing moments of joy and including things we create or do with others in a place we love, having a passion that makes us forget the pain, bringing a meaning to life, that comes from opening your heart, searching the invisible, giving your heart by offering your time, skills, compassion and unconditional love. All of these practices can help eliminate suffering. Peace and happiness depend on our emotions and our environment. Both are not permanent by themselves, must be learned to be reproduced and become a very significant part of our lives. When emotions and environment are modified into better conditions, suffering disappears to make some place for happiness. Pain becomes then an opportunity for achieving a new and healthier life and implementing a purpose in life. Being at peace with pain allows us to enjoy an extraordinary life in an extraordinary space.

In the final analysis, all of these suggested practices are performed most adequately when we find the internal resources to cease our incessant attachment to ourselves. No one can tell anyone else exactly how to do this. Our practice will always involve accepting some difficult facts about ourselves. The results of this process will always materialize if we work for them.

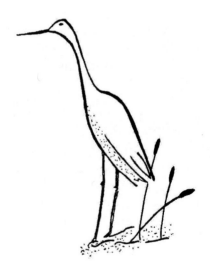

Endnotes

INTRODUCTION

1   Jackson, 2003, p. 301 and 357.
2   The singular first person pronoun "I" and corresponding words such as "my" or "mine" refer to Dr. Claude Roberto and her personal experiences with chronic pain. The plural "we" involves Dr. Claude Roberto and Dr. Paul Sussman.

CHAPTER 1

1   Nightmare is not simply a figure of speech when applied to chronic pain. Lawrence LeShan from the Institute of Applied Biology, described the universe perceived by the person with chronic pain as structurally identical with the universe of the nightmare. Nightmares, according to LeShan, possess three unvarying features: 1) Terrible things are being done and worse are being threatened. 2) We are helplessly under the control of outside forces. 3) We cannot predict when the ordeal will end. Information published in the Chronic Pain Association of Canada *Newsletter*, Fall 2001, Volume 5, Issue 3, p. 3; original source is unknown and used by the Chronic Pain Association of Canada with a note mentioning it was impossible to credit properly.
2   Hays, 1992, p. 3; Hunter, 1996, p. 2 – 3, 9.
3   Hunter, 1996, p. 4.
4   Nuland, 2003, p. 62.
5   Kalb, 2003, p. 48.
6   Dillard, 2002, p. 48.
7   Hunter, 1996, p. 2 – 3, 9.
8   Dillard, 2002, p. 3.

9   Hunter, 1996, p. 4 – 5, 9.
10 Dillard, 2002, p. 4.
11 Cottrell, 2001, p. 13 – 14.
12 Fishman, 2000, p. 108 – 109.
13 Fishman, 2000, p. 109 – 110.
14 Fishman, 2000, p. 66.
15 The McGill-Melzack Pain Questionnaire was developed in Canada to assess pain. It is based on identification by people in pain of words describing pain and placed in twenty groups. For additional information, see Wells, 1998, p. 102 – 103. See also Melzack, 1973, p. 42 – 43 where we took information to describe pain.
16 Kalb, 2003, p. 51.
17 Sussman and Ferguson, 1980.
18 Tunks, 1997, p. 176 – 177.
19 Margaret Caudill following Melzack, 1973, p. 21 – 24.
20 Fishman, 2000, p. 9.
21 Turk and Nash in Goleman and Gurin, 1993, p. 113 – 114; Caudill, 1995, p. 22 – 23, 34 – 35. See also Melzack, 1973, p. 83 – 92, 153 – 190.
22 Kalb, 2003, p. 46.
23 Caudill, 1995, p. 22 – 23, 34 – 35.
24 Kalb, 2003, p. 46.
25 Jetter, 1996, p. 69.
26 Kalb, 2003, p. 46.
27 For opinions on the connection mind-body, see also Turk and Nash in Goleman and Gurin, 1993, p. 115 – 117.
28 Kalb, 2003, p. 46, 51.
29 "Chronic pain-Signals in the brain," Chronic Pain Association of Canada *Newsletter*, Volume 6, Issue 4, Winter 2002 – 2003, p. 1 and 7 with information taken from Natalie Frazin, *Neuron*, 14 November 2002, Volume 36, p. 713 – 720.
30 Khalsa, 1999, p. 7, 12 – 13.
31 "The Management of chronic non-malignant pain," Chronic Pain Association of Canada, *Pain*, Volume 30, 1987, p. 1.
32 Kalb, 2003, p. 45; Chronic Pain Association of Canada *Newsletter*, Volume 7, Issue 3, Fall 2003, p. 4.
33 Chronic Pain Association of Canada *Newsletter*, Volume 7,

Issue 3, Fall 2003, p. 13.

34 Statistics provided by the Chronic Pain Association of Canada *Newsletter*, Volume 6, Issue 4, Winter 2002-2003, p. 1, 10 – 11.

35 Wells, 1998, p. XI – XII.

36 Wells, 1998, p. XII.

37 Figures taken from "The Management of chronic non-malignant pain," Chronic Pain Association of Canada, *Pain*, Volume 30, 1987, p. 2.

38 Stamatos, 2001 p. 237.

39 Figures provided by the Chronic Pain Association of Canada.

40 Khalsa, 1999, p. 21. See also Borde, 2004, p. 41.

41 Chronic Pain Association of Canada *Newsletter*, Volume 4, Issue 4, Winter 2000 – 2001, p. 7 and 10.

42 Springen, 2003, p. 54 – 61.

43 See Chronic Pain Association of Canada *Newsletter*, Volume 5, Issue 1, Spring 2001, p. 8 presenting information provided by the International Evidence-related Group for Neonatal Pain and published by Archives of Pediatric and Adolescent Medicine, 2001, 155, p. 173 – 180. For the time when a foetus can feel pain, see Dubé, 2000, p. 22.

44 Chronic Pain Association of Canada *Newsletter* , Volume 5, Issue 3, Fall 2001, p. 8.

45 Springen, 2003, p. 54 – 61; Chronic Pain Association of Canada *Newsletter*, Volume 3, Issue 2, Summer 1999, p. 7.

46 The quarterly newsletter published by the Chronic Pain Association of Canada owes much information on pediatric pain to research conducted by Dr. Patrick McGrath, Ph.D., Professor of Psychology, Pediatrics and Psychiatry, Dalhousie University, Psychologist Pediatric Pain Service, Grace Health Centre, Halifax, Nova Scotia, Canada.

47 Chronic Pain Association of Canada *Newsletter* , Volume 5, Issue 1, Spring 2001, p. 8 presenting information provided by the International Evidence-related Group for Neonatal Pain and published by *Archives of Pediatric and Adolescent Medicine*, 2001, 155, p. 173 – 180.

48 Bramham, 2004, p. D5.

49 For additional information on pediatric pain, see Dillard, 2002, p. 363 – 367.
50 Edwards, 2004, p. 2.
51 Edwards, 2004, p. 2.
52 Current figures from the Chronic Pain Association of Canada.
53 Current figures from the Chronic Pain Association of Canada.
54 All figures from the Chronic Pain Association of Canada.
55 Figures from the Chronic Pain Association of Canada.
56 "The management of chronic non-malignant pain," Chronic Pain Association of Canada, *Pain,* volume 30, 1987, p. 2.
57 Study under Dr. John Liebeskind, "The management of chronic non-malignant pain," Chronic Pain Association of Canada, *Pain,* Volume 30, 1987, p. 2 – 3.
58 Source: National Institutes of Health and Chronic Pain Association of Canada.
59 Siegel, 2001, p. 117.
60 Siegel, 2001, p. 228.
61 In "Manipulation and Mobilization of the Cervical Spine: A Systematic Review of Literature," *Spine,* 1998, p. 1753 – 1755 and table 5.
62 Dillard, 2002, p. 27.

CHAPTER 2

1 Hunter, 1996, p. 6 – 7, 21.
2 Fishman, 2000, p. 34.
3 Barnard, 1998, p. 61; Khalsa, 1999: "Aspirin can damage cartilage...Your cartilage...is like a sponge that keeps your bones from touching. But, to do that, it has to absorb water. Aspirin slows down this absorption, and makes your joints hurt even more," p. 122.
4 Historical notes taken from Fishman, 2000, p. 38 – 40.
5 *The Merck Manual,* 2003, R. Portenoy, p. 454.
6 "Acetaminophen is taken by mouth or suppository, and its effects generally last 4 to 6 hours. High doses can lead to liver damage, which may be irreversible. People with a liver disorder should use lower doses than usually taken. Whether

lower doses taken for a long time can harm the liver is less certain... Taking high doses for a long time may lead to kidney damage", *The Merck Manual*, 2003, R. Portenoy, p. 454.

[7] Barnard, 1998, p. 61; Marcus, 1994, p. 122; *The Merck Manual*, 2003, Portenoy, p. 454.

[8] Fishman, 2000, p. 41 – 42.

[9] Description of these procedures described by Dillard, 2002, p. 198 – 205.

[10] Fishman, 2000, p. 187.

[11] Fishman, 2000, p. 33.

[12] Turk and Nash, in Goleman, 1993, p. 118.

[13] Dillard, 2002, p. 49.

[14] Khalsa, 1999, p. 323 – 324.

[15] For additional information, see Saint-Arnaud, 2002, p. 408, 444 – 452.

[16] Ideas developed by Jackson, 2003, p. 5 who wrote that "it's almost as if pain flourishes on our diet of analgesics" and asked why we are "the most medicalized of societies" as well as "a culture in pain".

[17] Jackson, 2003, p. 8.

[18] "Too often, exaggerated concern about the addiction potential of opioids leads to undertreatment of pain and needless suffering. People with severe pain should not avoid opioids, and adequate doses should be taken as needed," *The Merck Manual*, 2003, Portenoy, p. 450, 452.

[19] Jackson, 2003, p. 7.

[20] Dossey, 1993, p. 135 – 137.

[21] Dossey, 1993, p. 137.

[22] Khalsa, 1999, p. 324.

[23] For additional information, see Saint-Arnaud, 2002, p.100 – 101.

[24] Saint-Arnaud, 2002, p. 88.

[25] Saint-Arnaud, 2002, p. 100.

[26] Fishman, 2000, p. 17.

[27] Fishman, 2000, p. 53.

[28] Source: 2003 conversation with Dr. Pierre Flor-Henry, Director, Alberta Hospital in Edmonton (Canada).

[29] Source: 2003 conversation with Dr. Pierre Flor-Henry,

Director, Alberta Hospital in Edmonton (Canada).

[30] Fishman, 2000, p. 33.
[31] Dossey, 1993, p. 200.
[32] Fishman, 2000, p. 33.
[33] Fishman, 2000, p. 33 – 34, 118; Jovey, 2002, p.1 – 2.
[34] Historical notes taken from Fishman, 2000, p. 37.
[35] Fishman, 2000, p. 187.
[36] Fishman, 2000, p. 187.
[37] Fishman, 2000, p. 111, 117.
[38] Saint-Arnaud lists other written sources concluding medications used as placebos cure up to 50% of cases, 2000, p. 35.
[39] Fishman, 2000, p. 117.
[40] Nuland, 2000, p. 268.
[41] Nuland, 2000, p. 269 – 271.
[42] Cited by Nuland, 2000, p. 271 – 272.
[43] Nuland also mentioned W. R. Houston, who in 1938 recognized that the placebo had always been the norm of medical practice, 2000, p. 272.
[44] Research on the link placebo-culture has been conducted by P. Lemoine, *Le Mystère du placebo*, Paris, Éditions Odile Jacob, 1996.
[45] Fishman, 2000, p. 119.
[46] Fishman, 2000. p. 119 – 120.
[47] Fishman, 2000, p. 120 – 121.
[48] Cited by Keene, 1998, p. 252.
[49] For additional information on clinical trials: http://content.health.msn.com/content/pages/13/66553.htm?z=1104_08201_8900
[50] Guidelines for research involving children are made available by the American Academy of Pediatrics at http://www.aap.org/policy/00655.html but unfortunately these are not mandatory even in the US.

CHAPTER 3

[1] Wells, Nown, 1998, p. 75.
[2] Dillard, 2002, p. 99.
[3] Dillard, 2002, p. 99.
[4] Khalsa, 1999, p. 99-100.

5 Khalsa, 1999, p. 101-102.
6 Adapted from Jackson, 1997, p. 41-43.
7 Historical notes from Facklam, 1996, p. 59-60.
8 Stamatos, 2001, p. 110.
9 Catty, 2002, p. 18.
10 Facklam, 1996, p. 61.
11 Khalsa, 1999, p. 90-91. Khalsa gives a map of the points on page 91.
12 Airey, *Healing hands*, 2003, p. 22-23.
13 Facklam, 1996, p. 61; Airey, *Healing hands*, 2003, p. 16-17.
14 Dillard, 2002, p. 150.
15 Facklam, 1996, p. 63.
16 Brown, 2001, p. 7.
17 Brown, 2001, p. 109-110.
18 Facklam, 1996, p. 65.
19 Khalsa, 1999, p. 106.
20 Dillard, 2002, p. 85.
21 Diamond and Schnell, 1996, p. 47.
22 Brody, 2000, p. 147.
23 Wells and Nown, 1998, p. 143-144.
24 Wells and Nown, 1998, p.143-144.
25 Wells and Nown, 1998, p. 145-146.
26 Facklam, 1996, p. 65.
27 For additional information: http://nioh.tripod.com/physio-therapy_scope_of_practice.htm; also http://www.gcau.org/carer/cx_physiotherapy.asp .
28 Khalsa, 1999, p. 107.
29 Dillard, 2002, p. 94.
30 For example, this is the definition given by the Webster Dictionary.
31 Definition taken from http://www.akta.org/.
32 Servan-Schreiber, 2003, p. 94-112.
33 Khalsa, 1999, p. 94-95.
34 Servan-Schreiber, 2003, p. 178.
35 Khalsa, 1999, p. 94.
36 Khalsa, 1999, p. 94.
37 Khalsa, 1999, p. 94.
38 Khalsa, 1999, p. 95-96.

[39] Servan-Schreiber, 2003, p. 180.
[40] Servan-Schreiber, 2003, p. 181.
[41] Rollot, 2003, p. 71-72.
[42] Barnard, 1998, p. 203.
[43] Dillard, 2002, p. 102.
[44] Corrections to bad habits taken from Marcus and Arbeiter, 1994, p.176-179.
[45] Khalsa, 1999, p. 111-112.
[46] Khalsa, 1999, p.112-113.
[47] See Facklam, 1996, p. 39.
[48] Rollot, 2003, p. 44.
[49] Marcus and Arbeiter, 1994, p. 188.
[50] Rollot, 2003, p. 53.
[51] Facklam, 1996, p. 40.
[52] Khalsa, 1999, p. 68-70.
[53] Barnard, 1998, p. 15; Khalsa, 1999, p. 64-68.
[54] Khalsa, 1999, p. 48-51.
[55] Inflammation description taken from Khalsa, 1999, p. 52-53.
[56] Facklam, 1996, p. 45.
[57] Barnard, 1998, p. 15, 54-56, 67, 84-87, 94-95; Khalsa, 1999, p. 56-63, 70-73; Dillard, 2002, p.137-147, 296.
[58] Barnard, 1998, p. 53.
[59] Barnard, 1998, p. 53.
[60] Dillard, 2002, p. 128-129.
[61] Barnard, 1998, p. 18-19, 42.
[62] Barnard, 1998, p. 55; Dillard, 2002, p. 129-135.
[63] Barnard, 1998, p. 52.
[64] Barnard, 1998, p. 49.

CHAPTER 4

[1] Khalsa, 1999, p. 173 – 174.
[2] Khalsa, 1999, p. 175.
[3] Jackson, 2003, p. 225.
[4] Cited from Jackson, 2003, p. 227.
[5] Caudill, 1995, p. 122.
[6] Wells and Nown, 1998, p. 98.
[7] Chronic pain syndrome, caused by pain, causes further pain.

This is known as the "cycle of pain" which kills the quality of life. It can be stopped by changing attitude according to Khalsa, 1999, p. 13.

[8] For details on recommended coping skills: see Khalsa, 1999, p. 182 – 183.

[9] Saint-Arnaud, 2002, p. 95.

[10] Khalsa, 1999, p.175.

[11] Khalsa, 1999, p. 175.

[12] Khalsa, 1999, p. 175.

[13] Khalsa, 1999, p. 176.

[14] Wells and Nown, 1998, p. 59.

[15] Caudill, 1995, p. 129.

[16] Khalsa, 1999, p. 177.

[17] Khalsa, 1999, p. 178.

[18] Khalsa, 1999, p. 178.

[19] For evidence and sources on benefits obtained from laughter, see Saint-Arnaud, 2002, p. 540 -562. Adults do not laugh as easily as children but anyone, young or older, can learn to laugh.

[20] For details on role of senses in fighting pain and for sources for this section on senses, see Saint-Arnaud, 2002, p. 112 – 130.

[21] Caudill, 1995, p. 112.

[22] Dillard, 2002, p. 107.

[23] Caudill, 1995, p. 39, 55.

[24] Wells and Nown, 1998, p. 78.

[25] Caudill, 1995, p. 33.

[26] Dossey, 1999, p. 19.

[27] Dossey, 1999, p. 19.

[28] For additional information on distant healing taken seriously, see Dossey, 1999, p. 14 – 15 who places this universal healing in what he calls "nonlocality."

[29] Dossey, 1999, p. 11.

[30] Caudill, 1995, p. 41.

[31] Caudill, 1995, p. 41.

[32] Khalsa, 1999, p. 190.

[33] For the physical benefits from breathing: Khalsa, 1999, p. 190 – 191.

[34] Hudson, 2003, p. 7.
[35] See http://www.here-and-now.org/VSI/Articles/TheoryMed/ theoryHow.htm p. 3 – 4; see also http://content.health.mns. com/content/article/72/81790.htm; see also http://www. buddhanet.net/tr20.htm, p. 1 – 12.
[37] Hudson, 2003, p. 25.
[38] Jackson, 2003, p. 13.
[39] Khalsa, 1999, p. 179.
[40] Khalsa, 1999, p. 179.
[41] Jackson, 2003, p. 20.
[42] Goleman and Gurin, 1993, p. 235 – 236.
[43] Goleman and Gurin, 1993, p. 270.
[44] Goleman and Gurin, 1993, p. 272.
[45] Goleman and Gurin, 1993, p. 304 – 305.
[46] Hunter, 1996, p. 21.
[47] Diamond and Schnell, 1996, p. 188 – 189.
[48] Diamond and Schnell, 1996, p. 189 – 190.
[50] See also Goleman and Gurin, 1993, p. 280.
[51] Caudill, 1995, p. 33.
[52] Goleman and Gurin, 1993, p. 286.
[53] Goleman and Gurin, 1993, p. 293.
[54] Khalsa, 1999, p. 186 – 187.
[55] http://www.americanyogaassociation.org/general.html, page 1.
[56] http://www.ronperfetti.com/specifics.html , p. 1 – 6.
[57] Hunter, 1996, p. 21.
[58] http://www'lifematters.com/taijin.html, p. 1.
[59] http://www.mtsu.ed/~jpurcell/Taichi/taichi.htm, p. 1.
[60] http://members.tripod.com/-zenist/taichi.hmtl, p. 1.
[61] http://www.ronperfetti.com/specifics.html p. 2.
[62] http://www.ronperfetti.com/specifics.html p. 6 – 11.
[63] http://www.mtsu.edu/~jpurcell/Taichi/taichi.htm , p.1 – 2.
[64] Khalsa, 1999, p. 37.
[65] Khalsa, 1999, p. 37 – 38.

CHAPTER 5

[1] Cited by Dillard, 2002, p. 21.
[2] Airey, *Healing energies*, 2003, p. 26 – 27.

4   For the importance of the number 7: Odoul, 2002, p. 131
    – 132.
5   For additional details, see Odoul, 2002, p. 133 – 249.
6   Hall, 2003, p. 20 – 21.
7   Lilly, 2003, p. 30.
8   Wells and Nown, 1998, p. 156.
9   Dillard, 2002, p. 153.
10 Wells and Nown, 1998, p. 157.
11 For details on feng shui: Airey, *Healing energies*, 2003, p. 44
    – 45.
12 Khalsa, 1999, p. 108; Lawrence, Rosch, Plowden, 1998, p. XX
    – XXII.
13 Khalsa, 1999, p. 109.
14 Lawrence, Rosch and Plowden, 1998, p. 84.
15 Airey, *Healing energies*, 2003, p. 48.
16 Washnis and Hricak, 1998, p. 200 – 201.
17 Lawrence, Rosch, Plowden, 1998, p. 2 – 19; Washnis and
    Hricak, 1998, p. 46 – 47.
18 Washnis and Hricak, 1998, p. 65.
19 Washnis and Hricak, 1998, p. 318.
20 Airey, *Healing energies*, 2003, p. 16 – 17.
21 Information taken from Airey, *Healing hands*, 2003, p. 32
    – 33.
22 Dillard, 2002, p. 166.
23 Airey, *Healing energies*, 2003, p. 46 – 47.
24 Khalsa, 1999, p. 132.
25 Airey, *Healing energies*, 2003, p. 24.
26 Khalsa, 1999, p. 133.
27 Facklam, 1996, p. 55.
28 acklam, 1996, p. 51 – 53.
29 Airey, *Healing energies*, 2003, p. 30 – 33; Lilly, 2003, p. 5
    – 63.
30 Khalsa, 1999, p. 107.
31 Airey, *Healing energies*, 2003, p. 40 – 41.
32 Dillard, 2002, p. 94.
33 Houdret, *Healing with flowers*, 2003, p. 6 – 7.
34 Information and table taken from Houdret, *Healing with
    flowers*, 2003, p. 22 – 23.

[35] Houdret, *Healing with flowers*, 2003, p. 12 – 13.
[36] Houdret, *Healing with flowers*, 2003, p. 8 – 9, 12 – 13, 49.
[37] Houdret, *Healing with herbs*, 2003, p. 12, 15.
[38] Houdret, *Healing with flowers*, 2003, p. 55 – 61.
[39] For additional details, see Lawless , 1994, p. 5 – 11.
[40] Jackson, 2003, p. 48.
[41] Evans, 2003, p. 58.
[42] Khalsa, 1999, p.114.
[43] Khalsa, 1999, p. 114 – 115.
[44] Source: www.chta.ca.

CHAPTER 6

[1] See also Ornish, 1998, p. 60 – 61.
[2] Formula adapted from Ornish, 1998, p. 60 – 61. This formula is also compatible with Siegel, 2001, p. 249, who believes the ill person does the loving, the healing and the teaching because these last three activities are included in connections.
[3] Candace Pert from the department of physiology and biophysics at Georgetown University Medical Center, Washington, D. C., citation published by Ornish, 1998.
[4] Joan Borysenko, specialist in anatomy and cellular biology, who cofounded the Mind/Body Institute at the Beth Israel Hospital, citation published by Ornish, 1998, p.193.
[5] Ornish, 1998, p. 223.
[6] Brody, 2000, p. 230-231.
[7] Ornish, 1998, p. 225.
[8] Brody, 1992, p. 45.
[9] Brody, 2000, p. 231.
[10] Brody, 2000, p. 231 – 232.
[11] Brody, 2000, p. 239 – 241.
[12] Keene, 1998, p. 25 – 26, 42 suggests other components to consider which will help you to define your needs in your relationships with therapists.
[13] This is an image often used and found at the beginning of the poem *The Divine Comedy* by Dante Alighieri when the poet was lost in a forest and needed a guide to put him back on the right way.

[14]   According to Korsch and Harding (1997, p. 103), timing
and dosage of information are important because "patients
should not be deceived by their doctors" and physicians
should "above all, do no harm." Korsch and Harding noted
also that "in medicine, truth is something we desire but
rarely acquire. Medicine is an imperfect art and nothing is
certain," p. 108. They agreed that "there is never just one
truth. There are a great many truths. There's a truth for the
doctor and a different truth for each and every patient," p.
108.

[15]   Our own personal experience confirms here the statement
from Korsch and Harding, 1998, p. 112, that talking about
everything is "a good way of judging the resiliency of the
relationship and of exploring what kinds of stresses it can
tolerate." This is true about any connections the person in
pain establishes.

[16]   Korsch and Harding mention that most doctors do not get
training with the human aspect of care, and believe that "
when physicians respond to patients exclusively as techni-
cians interested only in scientific aspects, they are not able
to achieve a complete therapeutic alliance," 1998, p. 162.
One of the activities currently undertaken by the Chronic
Pain Association of Canada is to introduce human contacts
between real persons in pain and medical students, in order
to make medical education more caring, and to introduce
students to struggles that people with chronic pain encounter in their lives.

[17]   Definition by Zolner, 2003, p. 8.

[18]   Zolner, 2003, p. 8.

[19]   Zolner, 2003, p. 8.

[20]   Definition of high road developed by Helliwell, 1999, p. 45
– 65.

[21]   Definitions of job and work taken from Helliwell, 1999, p. 9
– 10.

[22]   On the importance of interdependence, see Helliwell, 1999,
p. 42 – 46, 61 – 63.

[23]   Helliwell, 1999, p. 12.

[24]   Ornish, 1998, p. 121.

25 They follow the category presented by Ornish, 1998, p. 90 – 91, 100.
26 See Ornish, 1998, p. 79.
27 Citation taken from Ornish, 1998, p. 96.
28 Intuition is the "ability to make good decisions with little information" as defined by Joel Barker and mentioned by Helliwell, 1999, p. 291.
29 Adrienne, 1999, p. 239 – 240.
30 Ornish, 1998, p. 130 – 131.
31 Brody, 2000, p. 205.
32 Brody, 2000, p. 205 – 206 explaining the concept of "woundology" developed by Caroline Myss.
33 Ornish, 1998, p.33 – 35, conducted research on the way relations with parents have an impact on children's future health; love from parents and warm family relations in childhood reduces illnesses in future years.
34 St-Arnaud, 2002, p. 170.
35 St-Arnaud, 2002, p. 414 – 415.
36 Stanton, 2002, p. 57.
37 Ornish, 1998, p. 240.
38 Ornish, 1998, p. 200.
39 For additional information, see Stanton, 2002, p. 59 – 62.
40 For different opinions, see Siegel, 2001, p. 190 – 192, 196 – 197.
41 Adrienne, 1999, p. 84 – 90.
42 Dillard, 2002, p. 158.
43 Adrienne, 1999, p. 84 – 90, 207.
44 Adrienne, 1999, p. 84 – 90, 236.
45 Adrienne, 1999, p. 68 – 69.
46 Adrienne, 1999, p. 241, 242 and 250.
47 Adrienne, 1999, p. 239; for additional information on synchronicity, see Adrienne, 1999, p. 167 – 195.
48 For additional information on hints, see Helliwell, 1999, p. 88 – 90.
49 Adrienne, 1999, p. 206.
50 Adrienne, 1999, p. 78 – 81.
51 Millman, 2001, p. 102 – 103.
52 Adrienne, 1999, p. 207.

[53] Cited by Millman, 2001, p. 125.

CONCLUSION

[1] Pope John Paul, Apostolic Letter, *Salvifici Doloris*, 11 February 1984, http://www.vatican.va/holy_father/. Pope John Paul stated, on 12 November 2004 at a Vatican-sponsored conference on palliative care, that the use of painkillers for the dying was acceptable when appropriate (*Western Catholic Reporter*, 22 November 2004, p. 5).

[2] Ricard, 2003, p. 70 – 71.

[3] Ch'an Master Sheng-yen, 1999, p. 89 – 91.

[4] Ricard, 2003, p. 77 – 78.

[5] Dillard, 2002, p. 386 with a citation from Rachel Naomi Remen.

[6] Dillard, 2002, p. 386.

[7] Dillard, 2002, p. 389.

[8] See David B. Morris, *The Culture of Pain*, which shows the connection between pain and rites of passage, such as the secret pain rituals or the pain of childbirth exchanged for the responsibilities of parenting. According to Morris, "pain is a kind of tunnel through which one passes to a new stage of being."

[9] Robindranath Tagore, in Madeleen Dubois, 2004, p. 63.

[10] Benson, 1996.

[11] Hippocrates, *Precepts* I.

[12] Achterberg, Dossey, Kolkmeier, 1994, p. 9.

[13] Such as stated by Dr. Paul S. Sussman.

[14] Bernie Siegel, 2001, p. 9.

[15] 1978, p. 70 – 75.

[16] Vol. 1, *Timée*, 1953, p. 496 – 497.

[17] For these references to Socrates, see Plato, Volume 2, *Charmide*, 1955, p. 255 – 261.

[18] Socrates in Plato, Volume 2, *Alcibiade*, 1955, p. 243 – 247.

[19] 1946, preface.

[20] Vicinus, 1990, p. 264.

[21] Nightingale, 1946, p. 34.

[22] Nightingale, 1946, p. 48.

[23] Nightingale, 1946, p. 33 – 35, 48.

24 Nightingale, 1946, p. 49.

25 Joan Halifax in Carlson and Shield, 1989, p. 168 – 170.

26 Galland, 1997, p. 54.

27 See Galland, 1997, p. 55.

28 Lynn Andrews in Carlson and Shield, 1989, p. 42 – 43.

29 Elisabeth Küfler-Ross in Carlson and Shield, 1989, p. 129.

30 Cited by Galland, 1997, p. 105.

31 Galland, places the client-doctor relationship as the first pillar of healing and defines the qualities of a caring doctor, 1997, p. 108, p. 117 – 119.

32 This belief of a healing relationship is called "healing equation" and was developed by Norman Cousins in Carlson and Shield, 1989, p. 85 – 96.

33 Richard Moss in Carlson and Shield, 1989, p. 36 – 38.

34 Richard Moss in Carlson and Shield, 1989, p. 36 – 38.

35 In France people with migraines are likely to be diagnosed as having a liver disorder, in the United States with a vascular disorder and in England with a gastrointestinal problem. Medicine is not always an objective science. See Achterberg, Dossey, Kolkmeier, 1994, p. 11 for additional information.

36 Shakti Gawain in Carlson and Shield, 1989, p. 73.

37 Ideas presented by Bernie Siegel in Carlson and Shield, 1989, p. 7 – 9.

38 Serge Kahili King in Carlson and Shield, 1989, p. 29 – 30.

39 John E. Upledger in Carlson and Shield, 1989, p. 72.

40 Bernie Siegel in Carlson and Shield, 1989, p. 10.

41 Louise Hay in Carlson and Shield, 1989, p. 22 – 25.

42 Carlson and Shield, 1989, p. 33.

43 Carlson and Shield, 1989, p. 65.

44 Carlson and Shield, 1989, p. 63.

45 Martin Rossman in Carlson and Shield, 1989, p. 78.

46 Hugh Prather in Carlson and Shield, 1989, p. 15.

47 See Green, 2004, p. 216, 233.

48 Jack Schwarz in Carlson and Shield, 1989, p. 19.

49 Question proposed by D'Ansembourg, 2004, p. 98.

50 *Science*, November 2004, p. 113.

51 *Science*, November 2004, p. 111.

52 We agree with D'Ansembourg, 2004, p. 89 and Guy Corneau

cited by D'Ansembourg that being happy is usually not popular and natural in our society.

[53] Model taken from André, 2003, p. 240 – 241.

[54] André, 2003, p. 97.

[55] Cited by André, 2003, p. 152.

[56] André, 2003, p. 32.

[57] André, 2003, p. 165.

[58] Ricard, 2003, p. 30. Seneca committed a suicide in 65 AD and this action was for the Romans an active and positive way to end life.

[59] André, 2003, p. 17 – 18.

[60] André, 2003, p. 32.

[61] Cited by André, 2003, p. 60.

[62] Saint-Arnaud, 2002, p. 417.

[63] André, 2003, p. 122.

[64] See, for additional details, Saint-Arnaud, 2002, p. 538 – 571.

[65] Saint-Arnaud, 2002, p. 196.

[66] For details on benefits from music, see Saint-Arnaud, 2002, p. 119 – 122.

[67] André, 2003, p. 152.

[68] More details are found in Saint-Arnaud, 2002, p. 323.

[69] Saint-Arnaud, 2002, p. 324 – 326.

Significance of drawings:

The bear (p. 154) is the logo of the Chronic Pain Association of Canada. The heron is associatd with the book because it was a bird on the way to extinction, which managed to survive after many struggles.

Appendix

GLOSSARY OF TERMS

Acetaminophen: An over-the-counter pain reliever which reduces fever; the generic name for Tylenol®.

Acupressure: Apply pressure on painful points (such as along the spine) and massage these points for pain relief. Shiatsu is a form of massage based on acupressure.

Acupuncture: Insertion of fine needles into the body on meridian points for healing; a medical practice originating in China.

Acute pain: Sharp or severe pain which recedes over time.

Addiction: Compulsory dependence on a substance, even if the effects on the mind, the soul, the spirit or the body are negative. It is possible to be dependent on a medication without being addicted. We believe addiction needs not be a major concern as it is fairly rare among chronic pain clients according to statistics collected by the Chronic Pain Association of Canada.

Affirmation: Positive sayings that the ones in pain repeat to themselves. Affirmations are based on the idea that beliefs can have a positive effect on the body and affect perception of pain.

Alpha waves: Moderate brain waves (8-12 Hz) present

during relaxation and rest.

Altered state: Expression used when the mind, soul, spirit or body are in a different and momentary state. This condition can be induced during meditation, hypnotic trance or dream state.

Alternative medicine: Therapies employing treatments not depending on traditional western medicine. These therapies have generally not been scientifically tested.

Analgesic: Ability to relieve pain, usually referring to medications such as Tylenol®, Aspirin® or opioids.

Anesthetic: Substance, such as novocaine or ether, which produces local or general insensibility to pain.

Anesthetic therapies: Procedures such as medication infusion (see this term) into the spine or nerve block (see these terms).

Anticonvulsant: Medication that prevents, relieves or minimizes seizures.

Antidepressant: Medications used to treat depression. Opioids are not antidepressants.

Antioxidants: Compounds which inactivate dangerous chemical compounds called free radicals.

Aromatherapy: Healing therapy creating well-being from the use of odiferous substances such as essential oils. Different oils are connected to different conditions.

Arthritis: Pain and inflammation of the joints and soft tissues. Over 100 types of arthritis are identified. The four most common forms of arthritis are: osteoarthritis, gout, rheumatoid and systemic lupus. Cause is unknown, medical treatment is symptomatic.

Autogenic training: Relaxation technique focusing on feelings of heaviness and cultivating a sense of warmth in the limbs, combined with a focus on breathing.

Ayurvedic medicine: Ancient system of medicine from

India still followed in our times across the world and involving massage, meditation and herbs.

Behavior modification: System of positive and negative reinforcement influencing behavior.

Benzodiazepine: Pharmaceutical muscle relaxant with sedating properties.

Betawaves: Fast and short brain waves (≥12 Hz) developed during conscious mental activity.

Bioenergetics method: Therapy combining psychotherapy and movement to eliminate tension.

Biofeedback: Technique where the one in pain learns to become more aware of physical reactions to stress in order to better control these reactions. Biofeedback involves use of computers and sensors attached to parts of the body, for the client to see or hear muscle reactions. Providing information regarding physical body processes that ordinarily elude conscious awareness.

Block: Injecting a chemical to physically stop the transmission of pain signals in various parts of the body.

Bodywork: Physical therapies such as exercises, massages and bioenergetics.

Bone scan: Introduction of a radioactive dye into an artery to illuminate the blood flow to a bone and allow comparisons with the client's unaffected bones. A very safe and non painful procedure.

Breathwork: Therapy using breathing techniques for relief of tension, personal growth and awareness. It can induce an altered state in which insight and personal growth are facilitated.

C1 and C2: The top two vertebrae in the neck, also called Atlas and Axis. The top vertebra makes the transition between the neck and the head. These vertebrae must be touched with extreme care because they hold blood vessels going to and from the brain. They sometimes displaced as a result of whiplash.

CAT (computerized axial tomography) scan: Scan that displays computerized cross sections of the body, providing a three-dimensional picture of soft tissues such as the brain, lungs, liver and spleen.

Chakras: Sites, meaning wheel in Sanskrit, where energy is focused. Midline *chakras* govern specific activities and are also defined by colors allowing better visualization. These 7 points must be open in order to allow energy to flow for good functioning of the body, mind, spirit and soul. They can be opened with postures, psychotherapy and behavioral changes. The first *chakra* (red, at the base of the spine) is the root or connection to the earth, such as money; the second (orange, above the root chakra) is connected to passions, sexual energy, relationships, trust, control; the third *chakra* (yellow) is found on the solar plexus and has to do with personal power; the fourth (green, in the middle of the chest) is the centre of energy, a point of balance and the place of unconditional love; the fifth (blue, on the throat) is the location for creativity and communication; the sixth (purple, on the forehead) is the intuition place or psychic centre; the seventh (clear and transparent as a crystal) is located on top of the head and is the place for spiritual enlightenment.

Chi: Chinese word for the life forces of the body which are believed to be carried through the channels called meridians and *chakras*. If *chi* is blocked, the result is pain or disease.

Chinese medicine: Numerous healing techniques followed in China in the past and currently used across the world. This system includes acupuncture, massage and use of herbs.

Chiropractic: A manual manipulation of joints which allows alignment of the spine and can alleviate minor joint displacement. Uses active release technique which is a soft tissue technique breaking up with fingers adhesions (scar tissues) formed on injured muscles and tendons. These adhesions impair the oxygen and blood supply to the muscles.

Clairvoyance: Response to event or object without any known sensory contact (such as hearing or seeing).

Conventional medicine: Medicine commonly used in North America in contrast to alternative medicine.

Cranio-sacral therapy: Light massage involving manipulation of the bones in the skull and the sacrum.

Disability: Any restrictions or lack of ability to perform an activity in the manner or within the range considered normal for a human being (World Health Organization).

Distraction: Method used for pain relief by directing attention away from the pain, such as reading or talking.

Double effect: When the side effects of an analgesic increase vulnerability of the person in pain.

Electric stimulation: Also called TENS (Transcutaneous Electrical Nerve Stimulation). Therapy using brief electrical impulses to stimulate nerves through electrodes placed on the skin. Some stimulators can be permanently implanted.

EMG (electromyographic) biofeedback: Used to measure nerve damage. The EMG measures the speed of electric currents along nerve pathways. Abnormalities in the conduction of electricity indicate nerve damage. The procedure requires insertion of needles into the muscles along the nerve path. A rather painful test for the client.

Endorphins: Peptides in the body that act as natural opiates and raise one's pain threshold. The ones in pain do not build up tolerance to them. Exercise helps to increase output of endorphins. Synonymous with endorphins are the terms dynorphins and enkephalins.

Energy: Internal power or life force within a person which keeps the person alive and functioning. Also called *chi* in China or *prana* in India. See also *chakras*. Life energy circulates in the body by way of three channels: the masculine and solar one called *yang* in Chinese and the feminine and earth channel called *yin* also in Chinese. These energy channels merge with a third central channel at seven points on the spine called *chakras* in Sanskrit.

Epinephrine: Stress-response hormone that increases heart rate and blood pressure.

Family therapy: Psychotherapy which may help to ease pain or change reactions. Involves two or more persons.

Fascia: Band of connective tissue separating muscles and organs in the body. Chronic pain can be caused by injuries on the fascia becoming thick and hard. Normal fascia is loose and mobile, and allows joints and muscles to move. At the end of the muscle, fascia becomes a tendon connecting the muscle to the bone.

Fibromyalgia: Condition causing constant, unrelenting pain in the muscles, joints, ligaments and tendons. This condition involves various degrees of pain and is very difficult to treat medically. Diagnosed by presence of 15 out of 18 tender points on the body.

Fibrositis: See fibromyalgia. Term used in the 18th and 19th centuries replaced now by the word fibromyalgia.

Fight-or-flight response: When threatened, the body responds with an automatic secretion of stress hormones (epinephrine) preparing it to fight or run away.

Healing touch: Various physical therapies involving massages and exercises.

Heart-Centered Therapy: Psychological therapy healing the body, the mind, the soul and the spirit based on unconditional love.

Herbal therapy: Also called herbalism. This therapy is based on use of herbs for relief of pain. Herbs can be massaged into the skin, used in a bath, taken as a capsule, ingested by a tea or infusion.

Hippocrates: Greek physician born in 460 B.C and regarded as the Father of Medicine. His Hippocratic oath is taken by all physicians today.

Homeopathy: A therapy very popular in Europe and not well accepted in Northern America. It is based on the principle that "like cures like". A substance causing a medical symptom in a healthy person will cure the same symptoms in a sick person and will thus force the immune system to prevent disease.

Hydrotherapy: Therapy using water.

Hypnosis: State of consciousness where the unconscious mind is present and the person is open to suggestions. Hypnosis can be self-induced through relaxation or concentration on own breathing and can appear with numerous other techniques. It occurs normally in every person just before falling into sleep, and can block or transform or reduce pain.

Hypnotic trance state: State induced by hypnosis.

Ibuprofen: Generic name for Motrin® and Advil®. Often used to control the pain of arthritis.

Idiopathic: Of unknown origin.

Imagery: Use of mental images produced by memory or imagination. See visualization.

Inflammation: A major cause of chronic pain. It is a natural part of body's response to injury. Chronic inflammation can become the pathology of certain diseases.

Infusion: Medication flowing by gravity into a vein. Intravenous infusion is different from injection by syringe.

Intrathecal infusion: Surgically implanted pump that delivers pain medication directly to the local area, usually the spine.

Karma: Law of cause and effect. It is believed the effect of past karma has an impact on current life. Present happiness or suffering would be the result of past actions or karma.

Kinesiology: Study of muscles and their relation to movement.

Lumbago: Non-medical term meaning pain in the back.

Lumbar spine: The 5 vertebrae between the thoracic vertebrae and the lumbosacral area.

Magnetic therapy: Use of magnets to treat physical conditions, including pain.

Meditation: Different practices employed to relax the mind, soul, spirit and body, usually focusing on one thing such as breath, or an image or a word or short phrase. However several other forms of meditation can be practiced and they include tai chi involving movement, visualization with concentration on a mental image, loving kindness meditation requesting compassion for the universe, and transformative meditation changing negative emotions into positive energies.

Mind-body medicine: Therapies, such as meditation, using the mind to relax muscles and to decrease or relieve pain in the body.

Mindfulness: A classification of meditation practice (see transcendental meditation for other major classification) also known as *vipassana* or insight meditation. When thoughts or feelings come up in the mind, they are noted and observed as they occur. This notion of thoughts coming and going may give the feeling to be less caught up in them and this technique makes it possible to see what is actually on the mind.

Modality-oriented clinic: Health care facility offering a specific type of treatment and not providing comprehensive assessment and treatment, for example an acupuncture clinic or biofeedback clinic.

Morphine: A principal element of opium and a commonly used analgesic.

MRI (magnetic resonance imaging): Noninvasive test using magnetic and radio waves to display computer-generated sectional images of the body and its internal structure. This imaging technique uses magnetic energy without x-ray exposure.

Multidisciplinary pain centre: Organization of health care professionals and basic scientists which includes research, teaching and client care related to acute and chronic pain. Ideally a pain centre is a component of a medical school or teaching hospital. Health care services are integrated and based on multidisciplinary assessment and management of the client.

Multidisciplinary pain clinic: Facility staffed by physicians of different specialties and other health care providers who specialize in the diagnosis and management of people with pain.

Muscle knot: Hard mass formed by one or several muscles when muscles freeze in contraction without relaxing. The knot puts pressure on blood vessels and lymphatic veins which then stop functioning properly. Consequently nutrition and toxin elimination are denied to the muscle.

Muscles related to back pain: Include abdominal muscles, adductor, gluteus maximus, gluteus medius, hamstrings, latissimus dorsi, piriformis, psoas, quadratus lumborum, quadriceps, sacrospinalis, tensor fascia lata.

Muscle spasm: Very painful condition, very difficult to treat, where a muscle or several muscles contract involuntarily. This creates pain, stiffness, distortion and prevents the nerve energy to flow in the body. It can also pull the joints out of place. Massages help to fight muscle spasms. Muscle spasms occur when the muscle is stretched or overworked, causing it to contract. Several things happen during a muscle spasm: the spasm activity releases lactic acid into the immediate area; as the muscle works and works through a spasm, it releases much lactic acid which the non increased blood flow does not carry away to the liver to break it down. Because of the buildup of lactic acid, the muscle has no chance to relax and recover. The acid irritates the affected muscles and the surrounding area. In addition, other muscles around the injured area work harder to compensate for the muscles locked in a spasm. Finally the injured muscle returns over and over to spasms because it begins to remember spasms as a normal state.

Muscle tension: Condition where the muscles are contracted.

Myofascial pain: Muscle and soft tissue referred pain caused by trigger points. This type of pain includes muscle spasms, swelling of tissue and/or injured bones. Myofascial pain is often aggravated by stress.

Myofascial release: Relaxing the fascia (sheath) around a muscle by massages and gentle movements.

Narcotic: Synonym of opioid or opiates, used as analgesics, and chemically related to opium. These analgesics are available in two types, long acting and short acting.

Naturopathy: This therapy is based on the premises that the body can heal itself and the ones in pain must be active in taking care of their health. It emphasizes preventive measures. Naturopaths use nutrition, herbalism, psychology, homeopathy, traditional Chinese medicine and other physical therapies.

Nerve block: Injection of an anesthetic into a nerve site for pain relief.

Neuralgia: Pain along the course of a nerve.

Neuritis: Inflammation of a nerve, often accompanied by edema of the nerve.

Neuron: A nerve cell, the functional unit of the nervous system.

Neuropathic pain: Deep, burning, intense pain, caused by injury to or prolonged activation of peripheral nociceptors and central nociceptive pathways. This pain is very difficult to treat and it is increased by physical activity, deep massages, emotions and environmental conditions.

Neurostimulatory procedures: Procedures such as electric stimulation (see these terms) or acupuncture (see this term).

Neurotransmitter: Any of several chemical substances, such as epinephrine, released by nerve cells that act upon other nerve cells, or muscles, or glands, and transmitting nerve impulses.

Nonprescription: Same meaning as over-the-counter (OTC). Medication which can be bought without a doctor's prescription.

NSAIDs (non-steroidal anti-inflammatory medications): Pharmaceutical substances, such as ibuprofen or aspirin, that act like (but are not) steroids and reduce inflammation.

Occupational therapy: Therapy where the ones in pain learn ways to regain independence and physical ability at work and home.

Opiate or opioid: Any opium-like substance, whether

natural (such as endorphins) or synthetic (such as metha-done). See also narcotic. Opiate is any medication made from opium.

Opioid phobia: Fear of use of opioids.

Osteopathy: System of medicine based on the belief that structural defects lead to disease and can be treated by manipulation of the body, especially the spine.

Pain: Unpleasant sensory and emotional experience, typi-cally associated with actual or potential tissue damage or described in terms of such damage. Pain becomes chronic when it persists beyond the usual course of an acute illness or injury (usually beyond 3 or 6 months), associated with a pattern of recurrence, or associated with a chronic patho-logical process. See chapter 1.

Pain clinic: Health care facility focusing on the diagno-sis and management of people with pain. It may special-ize in specific diagnoses or in pains related to a specific region of the body. It can house research. A single physi-cian functioning within a complex health care institution which offers appropriate consultative and therapeutic ser-vices could qualify as a pain clinic if pain clients are suit-ably assessed and managed. The absence of interdisciplin-ary assessment and management distinguishes this type of facility from a multidisciplinary pain centre or clinic.

Pain management plan: List of activities, therapies and strategies planned to relieve pain.

Pain threshold: Level at which a person becomes aware of pain. This level is often referred to as either low or high, depending on the location on the scale when someone becomes aware of pain. It is different from pain tolerance.

Pain tolerance: Amount of pain a person is able to with-stand before being unable to function. This amount differs for everyone.

Palliative care: Medical and/or tertiary care during the final 3 months of life after active treatment has stopped and supportive ones are in place.

PCA (patient-controlled analgesia): Intravenous device that allows the client to deliver his/her own pain medication as needed, at predetermined maximum levels and at maximum intervals.

Peripheral nerves: Sensory nerves throughout the body, excluding the ones in the spinal cord and brain.

Personal transformation: Changing oneself throughout a process having an impact on the body, mind, soul, and spirit.

Physical therapy or **physiotherapy**: Health profession treating pain in muscles, nerves, tendons, joints, bones with exercises, electrical stimulation, massage, hot or cold pads and electrical devices. Often is done post-surgery and may include learning to walk or perform other daily activities.

Placebo: Inert formulation administered in place of an actual pharmaceutical or recognized formulation. Ethically and legally, the possibility of receiving placebo medication must be done with the consent of the client, and is normally done primarily in approved medical trials. Different from placebo effect.

Placebo effect: It occurs when clients report the desired effect of a medication or alternative treatment on trial, when they are actually receiving an inert medication or therapy. This occurs due to the clients' belief that proper treatment is being administered.

Prana: In Ayurvedic medicine, life force taken into the body by breathing. Similar to the Chinese *chi*.

Pranyama: Breathing exercises to relax the mind and calm the body.

Prayer: Spiritual exercise offering praise to a divine power, and asking for forgiveness and assistance in daily or life challenges. See chapter 4.

Progressive muscle relaxation: Relaxation technique combined with a passive attitude or voice guidance, where the client recognizes muscle contractions and subsequently releases them to achieve a deep state of muscular relaxation.

Psychosomatic: Physical symptoms with an emotional or psychological basis.

Psychotherapy: Numerous types of therapy integrating cognitive methods (such as relaxation, hypnosis or biofeedback) and interior forces to heal the body, the mind, the soul and the spirit. See chapter 4.

Reflexology: Therapy when pressure is applied on specific points on the hands or feet to improve the condition of specific parts of the body said to be connected to these pressure points.

Reiki: Healing system of Japanese origin, redirecting energy in the body with gentle hand placements on the body. Spiritual in origin and nature of training.

Relaxation techniques: Healing system removing effects of stress by reducing anxiety. See progressive muscle relaxation, on this glossary, which is one component of these techniques.

Sacroiliac syndrome: Pain caused by damage to the sacroiliac joint located between the hip joints and the spine.

Sciatica: Sharp pain radiating down the sciatic nerve on the outer edge of the leg caused by compression of the nerve.

Shiastu massage: Japanese massage technique of acupressure or acupuncture points that balances energy throughout the body.

Side effect: Symptom resulting from the use of medications, mostly undesirable and often unavoidable. They are tried to be kept to a minimum through dosage control and adjunct therapy.

Spirituality: Belief system based on the soul or influenced by a superior force, such the Holy Spirit or other divinity.

Steroid: One of a large group of fat-soluble organic compounds that help to return or improve function, often involve adrenal glands, and are designed for short term therapy if possible. Complicated treatment presents potential severe and long-lasting side effects.

Strained muscle: Overstretching of a muscle which can cause severe pain.

Stress management: Various techniques undertaken to prevent and treat the physical and emotional effects of stress. Training is often provided on request to employers and psychotherapists.

Suggestion: Idea or feeling which is introduced often into the mind as a healing tool.

Syndrome: Collection of symptoms often causing an undesirable effect. A chronic pain syndrome includes inability to work, family problems, depression and many other issues added to pain. A syndrome has no known pathology, as does the term disease.

Swedish massage: Form of bodywork using strokes to increase blood and lymph circulation.

Tai chi: Gentle Chinese martial art involving dance movements and very effective for stress and pain relief. Tai chi promotes proper circulation of energy (*chi*) throughout the body.

Temporomandibular joint disorder (TMJ): Pain and dysfunction in the joint located at the front of the ear, connecting the upper and lower jaws. The pain can radiate to include the entire head and neck. When the disc in the joint does not function well, it limits the opening of the jaw and mouth. This disorder can be caused by stress, arthritis or damage to the bone or soft tissue around the joint. It can also cause chronic grinding and wear of teeth, pain in the maxillary bone, tinnitus and light headedness. Insurance coverage for TMJ dysfunction is minimal if any. Therapy includes massages, relaxation, exercises, dental treatment and sometimes surgery.

TENS: See electric stimulation.

Therapeutic touch: Adjustment and balancing of a person's energy field involving the placement of hands on various positions on the body.

Tolerance: The decreasing effect of a medication of the same dose, and/ or need to increase the dose to maintain the same effect. Often occurs with opioids and sedatives.

Tranquilizer: Sedative used to decrease anxiety.

Transcendental: Ability to experience yourself psychologically at several ages and/or places at once.

Transcendental meditation: Meditation with attention focused on something, usually the sensation of breath leaving and entering the body or chanting of a mantra (special sound or phrase repeated silently).

Trigger point: Hard and small nodules, in tightly knotted muscle tissue, caused by accumulation of scar tissue which prevents muscles from moving as freely as needed above and below each other.

Trigger point therapy: Application of pressure on tender trigger points in the muscles to relieve pain and tension. Can be accomplished by active release technique (see chiropractic).

Unconscious mind: Activity of a person's mind (such as

fear or memories) taking place without awareness or control by the person.

Visualization: Synonym of imagery. The mind concentrates on a pleasant mental image in order to achieve physical and mental healing by changing the perception of pain.

Whiplash: Act to straining muscles usually in the neck. Occurs when one car is rear-ended by another, and the head snaps back forward and is then forced quickly ahead due to the impact of the crash.

Yin and **yang**: In ancient Chinese philosophy they are the two complementing energy forces. *Yin* is dark and feminine, *yang* is bright and masculine. These forces interact and influence all aspects of life; the ideal is to balance them in order to prevent or cure disease.

Yoga: Exercise system, usually gentle, consisting of stretching movements very helpful in healing. Numerous forms of yoga include *hatha* (balanced workout with emphasis on poses), *ashtanga* (fast-paced vigorous workout also known as power or dynamic yoga), *Iyengar* (exercises customized to your needs, also called furniture yoga), *bikram* (hot yoga at 40 C with sweating to cleanse body toxins), *kripalu* (meditation in motion) and *kundalini* (spiritual experience described as an exercise of awareness).

Yoga therapy: Use of yoga positions to reduce stress (often caused by pain originating from mental, spiritual and physical problems). Also useful for day to day reduction of stress and for maintaining balance in life.

Note: The authors experienced personally most treatments defined in this appendix.

Selected sources: http://www.garyflegal.com/glossary.htm
    Chronic Pain Association of Canada
    International Association for the Study of Pain
    Facklam, Howard, 1996.
    Fishman, Scott, 2000.
    Khalsa, Dharma Singh with Cameron Stauth, 1999.
    John M. Stamatos, 2001.

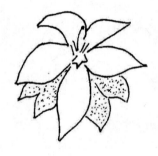

Bibliography

Achterberg, Jeanne, Dossey, Barbara, Kolkmeier, Leslie, *Rituals of healing, using imagery for health and wellness*, New York: Bantam Books, 1994.

Adrienne, Carol, *Votre Mission de Vie*, Montréal: Les Éditions du Roseau, 1999.

Airey, Raje, *Healing energies, Using the powers of nature to heal mind, body and spirit*, London: Hermes House, 2003 (2002).

Airey, Raje, *Healing hands, a concise guide to the therapeutic power of touch*, London: Hermes House, 2003 (2002).

American Society of Law, Medicine and Ethics, "Pain Relief Act," *Journal of Law, Medicine & Ethics*, Volume 24 (4), Winter 1996, p. 317 – 318.

André, Christophe, *Vivre heureux, Psychologie du bonheur*, Paris: Éditions France Loisirs, 2003.

Barnard, Neal and Raymond, Jennifer, *Foods that Fight Pain, Revolutionary New Strategies for Maximum Pain Relief*, New York: Harmony Books, 1998.

Barritt, Evelyn R., *Florence Nightingale, her Wit and Wisdom*, New York: Peter Pauper Press, 1975.

Bedard, Jim, *Lotus in the Fire, The Healing Power of Zen*, Boston: Shambhala, 1999.

Bensaid, Catherine, *La musique des anges, S'ouvrir au milieu de soi*, Paris: Éditions France Loisirs, 2003.

Benson, Herbert, *The Relaxation Response*, New York: William Morrow, 1975.

Benson, Herbert with Marg Stark, *Timeless Healing, the Power and Biology of Belief*, New York: Scribner, 1996.

Bernstein, Douglas A. and Borkovec, Thomas D., *Progressive Relaxation Training, A Manual for the Helping Professions*,

Champaign: Research Press, 1973.

Borde, Valérie, *L'Actualité*, 2004, p. 41.

Bowers, Kenneth S., *Hypnosis for the Seriously Curious*, New York: W. W. Norton and Company, 1976.

Bramham, Daphne, "Have kids been guinea pigs?", *Edmonton Journal*, February 8, 2004, p. D5.

Brody, Howard, *The Healer's Power*, New Haven and London: Yale University Press, 1992.

Brody, Howard and Brody, Daralyn, *The Placebo Response, How You Can Release The Body's Inner Pharmacy for Better Health*, New York: Harper Collins, 2000.

Brown, Whichello Denise, *Réflexologie par les mains*, Laval (Québec) : Modus Vivendi, 2001.

Burack, Marsha, *Reiki – Healing Yourself and Others*, Encinitas : Lo Ro Productions, 1995.

Canadian Pain Society, "Use of Opioid Analgesics for the Treatment of Chronic Non-Cancer Pain, A Consensus Statement and Guidelines," *Pain Res Manage*, Volume 3, No 4, Winter 1998, p. 197 – 208.

Carlson, Richard and Shield, Benjamin (Editors), *Healers on Healing*, New York : Penguin Putnam Inc., 1989.

Catty, Suzanne, Lacombe, Jean, Muzard, Pascal, Paré, Véronique, Poirier, Francine, *Aux petits maux les nouveaux remèdes*, Québec Loisirs, 2002.

Caudill, Margaret A., *Managing Pain before it Manages You*, New York: Guilford Press, 1995.

Ch'an Master Sheng-yen, *Complete Enlightenment*, Boston: Shambhala Publications, 1999.

Chronic Pain Association of Canada (CPAC), *Newsletter* and *Fact Sheet*, Edmonton, 1985-2003.

Chronic Pain Association of Canada, "The Management of Chronic Non-Malignant Pain," *Pain*, Volume 30, 1987, p. 1 – 9.

Cobb, Kevin, *Men's Fitness Magazine's Complete Guide to Health and Well-Being*, New York: Harper Collins, 1996.

Coombs, Ann, *The Living Workplace, Soul, Spirit, and Success in the 21th Century*, Toronto: Harper Collins, 2001.

Corneau, Guy, *La Guérison du Coeur, Nos souffrances ont-elles un *sens?*, Les Éditions de l'Homme, 2000.

Cottrell, Kate, "Conquering Chronic Pain," *Healthy Woman*, October-November 2001, p. 13 – 14.

D'Ansembourg, Thomas, *Être heureux, ce n'est pas nécessairement confortable*, Les Éditions de l'Homme, 2004.

Davidson, Jonathan R.T. and Connor, Kathryn M., *Herbs for the mind: what science tells us about nature's remedies for depression, stress, memory loss and insomnia*, New York: The Guilford Press, 2000.

Dean, Ornish, *Love and Survival, the Scientific Basis for the Healing Power of Intimacy*, New York: Harper Collins Publishers, 1998.

De Saint-Exupéry, Antoine, *The Little Prince*, translated by Irene Testot-Ferry, Ware: Wordsworth Classics, 1995.

Diamond, Marilyn and Schnell, Donald Burton, *Fitonics for Life*, New York: Avon Books, 1996.

Dienstfrey, Harris, *Where the Mind Meets the Body, Type A, the Relaxation Response, Psychoneuroimmunology, Biofeedback, Neuropeptides, Hypnosis, Imagery and the Search for the Mind's Effect on Physical Health*, New York: Harper Collins, 1991.

Dillard, James N. with Leigh Ann Hirschman, *The Chronic Pain Solution: Your Personal Path to Pain Relief, The Comprehensive, Step-by-Step Guide to Choosing the Best of Alternative and Conventional Medicine*, New York: Bantam Books, 2002.

Dossey, Larry, *Be Careful What You Pray for...You Just Might Get it: What We Can Do about the Unintentional Effects of our Thoughts, Prayers and Wishes*, New York: Harper Collins, 1997.

Dossey, Larry, *Healing Words: The Power of Prayer and the Practice of Medicine*, New York: Harper Collins, 1993.

Dossey, Larry, *Prayer is Good Medicine: How to Reap the Healing Benefits of Prayer*, San Francisco: Harper Collins, 1996.

Dubé, Catherine, "Enfants et douleur: La fin des larmes," *Québec Science*, April 2000, p. 22 – 24.

Dubois, Madeleene, *Communiquer avec son âme*, Éditions Quebecor, 2004.

Duncan, Barry, Miller, Scott, Sparks, Jacqueline, "Exposing the Mythmakers," *Networker*, March-April 2000, p. 24 – 53.

Editors of Time-Life Books, *The Medical Advisor, The Complete Guide to Alternative and Conventional Treatments*, Alexandria, Virginia: Time Life, Second Edition, 2000.

Edwards, Robert R., *Age-associated differences in pain responses and pain modulation: clinical relevance and implications*, Syllabus, Session 316, May 6-9, 2004, Vancouver, p. 2.

Egoscue, Pete and Gittines, Roger, *Pain Free, a Revolutionary Method for Stopping Chronic Pain*, New York: Bantam Book, 1998.

Engel, Cindy, *Wild Health, How animals keep themselves well and what we can learn from them*, New York: Houghton Mifflin Company, 2002.

Evans, Mark, *Healing with aromatherapy, A concise guide to using essential oils for health, harmony and happiness*, London: Hermes House, 2003 (2002).

Facklam, Howard, *Alternative Medicine, cures or myths?*, New York: Twenty-First Century Books, 1996.

Fisher, Stanley with James Ellison, *Discovering the power of Self-Hypnosis, The Simple, Natural Mind-Body Approach to Change and Healing*, New York: Newmarket Press, 2000 (1991).

Fishman, Scott with Lisa Berger, *The War on Pain: How Breakthroughs in the New Field of Pain Medicine Are Turning the Tide Against Suffering*, New York: Harper Collins, 2000.

Fleetwood, Jenni, *Healing with food, A concise guide to using the therapeutic properties of food to stay healthy and fight infection*, London: Hermes House, 2003 (2002).

Flemons, Douglas, "The Tao of Therapy," *Psychotherapy Networker*, May-June 2004, p. 44 – 47, 68.

Frankl, Viktor F., *Man's Search for Meaning*, New York: Pocket Books, 1963.

Galland, Leo, *The Four Pillar of Healing, How the New Integrated Medicine – the Best of Conventional and Alternative Approaches – Can Cure You*, New York: Random House, 1997.

Garofalo, John Paul and LaVonne Wesley, A., "Research Diagnostic Criteria for Temporomandibular Disorders: Reflection of the Physical-Psychological Interface," *American Pain Society Bulletin*, May-June 1997, p. 4 – 16.

Gelb, Harold and Siegel, Paula M., *Killing Pain without Prescription*,

New York: Barnes and Noble Books, 1982 (1980).

George, Lianne, "Are you ready for your mental makeover? Got a problem? We've got a pill," *Maclean's,* June 2005, p. 32 – 35.

George, Mike, *Discover Inner Peace, A Guide to Spiritual Well-Being,* San Francisco: Chronicle Books, 2000.

Goldstein, Joseph and Kornfield, Jack, *Seeking the Heart of Wisdom, The Path of Insight Meditation,* Boston: Shambala Dragon Editions, 1987.

Goleman, Daniel and Gurin, Joel, *Mind Body Medicine, How to Use your Mind for Better Health,* New York: Consumer Reports Books, 1993.

Green, Penelope, "Dirty Pretty Things," *Vogue,* February 2004, p. 216, 233.

Greenwood, Michael and Nunn, Peter, *Paradox and Healing, A book about medicine, mythology and transformation,* Victoria (Canada): Paradox Publishers, 1994.

Hagen, Neil A., "Opioids for Chronic Nonmalignant Pain: Shaping a National Health Care Agenda through Practice Guidelines," *Pain Res Manage,* Volume 3, No 4, Winter 1998, p. 193 – 196.

Hall, Doriel, *Healing with yoga, A holistic way to unite body and mind for greater wellbeing and serenity,* London: Hermes House, 2003 (2002).

Hawkins, Mary F., *Health Talk: How to Communicate with your Doctor,* Toronto: Macmillan Canada, 2000.

Hays, Helen, "Acute and Chronic Pain: What can we do?", *Trends in Bioethics,* March 1992, p. 3-7.

Helliwell, Tanis, *Take your Soul to Work. Transform your Life and Work,* Random House of Canada, 1999.

Hippocrate, *Des Lieux dans l'homme,* tome XIII, Paris: Les Belles Lettres, 1978.

Homer, *The Odyssey,* translated into English by Allen Mandelbaum, Berkeley and Los Angeles: University of California Press, 1990.

Houdret, Jessica, *Healing with flowers, A concise guide to using flowers to balance the mind, body and emotions,* London : Hermes House, 2003 (2002).

Houdret, Jessica, *Healing with herbs, A concise guide to natural her-*

bal remedies for everyday ailments, London : Hermes House, 2003 (2002).

Huddleston, John, *The Earth is but one country*, New Delhi (India) : Baha'i Publishing Trust, 1996 (1976).

Hudson, John, *Healing with meditation, A concise guide to clearing, focusing and calming the mind*, London: Hermes House, 2003 (2002).

Hunter, Marlene E., *Making Peace with Chronic Pain, A Whole-Life Strategy*, New York: Brunner/Mazel, Inc., 1996.

Inglis, Brian, *Natural Medicine*, London: Collins, 1979.

Jackson, Judith, *The Magic of Well-Being*, Montreal: Reader's Digest, 1997.

Jackson, Marni, *Pain: The Fifth Vital Sign*, Random House Canada, 2002.

Jackson, Marni, *Pain, the science and culture of why we hurt*, Toronto: Vintage Canada, 2003.

Jetter, Alexis, "The End of Pain", *Health*, September 1996, p. 67 – 72.

Jovey, Roman D. (Editor), *Managing Pain, The Canadian Healthcare Professional's Reference*, Toronto: Healthcare & Financial Publishing, Rogers Media, 2002.

Jovey, R.D., Ennis, J., Gardner-Nix, J., Goldman, B., Hays, H., Lynch, M., Moulin, D., "Use of opioid analgesics for the treatment of chronic noncancer pain – A consensus statement and guidelines from the Canadian Pain Society, 2002," *Pain Research and Management*, reprinted from *Pain Res Manage* 2003; 8 (Suppl A): 1A – 14A.

Jung, Carl Gustav, *L'Énergie psychique*, Genève: Librairie de l'Université; Paris: Buchet-Chastel, 1956.

Jung, Carl Gustav, *Les Types psychologiques*, Genève: Librairie de l'Université, Georg & Cie, S. A., 1968.

Kalb, Claudia, "A New Look at Pain," *Newsweek*, 19 May 2003, p. 44 – 52.

Keene, Nancy, *Working with your Doctor, Getting the Healthcare you Deserve*, Sebastopol, California : O'Reilly, 1998.

Kenyon, Julian, *Acupressure Techniques, A Self-Help Guide*, Wellinborough (England): Thorsons, 1987.

Khalsa, Dharma Singh with Cameron Stauth, *The Pain Cure, the proven medical program that helps end your chronic pain,* New York: Time Warner Company, 1999.

King, Serge, *Imagineering for Health,* Wheaton: Theosophical Publishing House, 1994 (1981).

Korsch, Barbara and Harding, Caroline, *The Intelligent Patient's Guide to the Doctor-Patient Relationship, Learning how to talk so your doctor will listen,* New York: Oxford University Press, 1997.

Lantos, John D., *Do We Still Need Doctors?,* New York: Routledge, 1997.

Law, Jaclyn, "Yoga your way," *Châtelaine,* July 2003, p. 101 – 104.

Lawless. Julia, *Aromatherapy and the Mind, An Exploration into the Psychological and Emotional Effects of Essential Oils,* London: Thorsons, 1994.

Lawrence, Ron, Rosch, Paul, Plowden, Judith, *Magnet Therapy, The Pain Cure Alternative,* Rocklin: Prima Publishing, 1998.

Lilly, Simon, *Healing with crystals, A concise guide to using crystals for health, harmony and happiness,* London: Hermes House, 2003 (2002).

Lowry, Lois, *The Giver,* New York: Bantam, 1993.

Lynch, Mary, *Surviving your Personal Injuries Claim and Litigation: A Guidebook,* Halifax, 2003.

Madorsky, Rachel, *Create your Own Destiny! Spiritual Path to Success,* Northbrook (IL): Avanty House, 2003.

Mailis-Gagnon, Angela and Israelson, David, *Beyond Pain: making the mind-body connection,* Toronto: Penguin Books, 2003.

Marcus, Norman J. and Arbeiter, Jean S., *Freedom from Chronic Pain, The Breakthrough Method of Pain Relief Based on the New York Pain Treatment Program at Lenox Hill Hospital,* New York: Simon & Schuster, 1994.

Melzack, Ronald, *The Puzzle of Pain,* Harmondsworth: Penguin Education, 1973.

Melzack, Ronald, "The Tragedy of Needless Pain," *Scientific American,* 1993, p. 45 – 51.

Merskey, Harold and Teasell, Robert W., "The Disparagement of pain: Social Influences on Medical Thinking," *Pain Res Manage,* Volume 5, No 4, Winter 2000, p. 259 – 270.

Millman, Dan, *Accomplir sa Mission, Réponses simples à des questions fondamentales*, Montréal: Éditions du Roseau, 2001 (2000, Dan Millman).

Modus Vivendi, *Le Bonheur, un jour à la fois*, Québec Loisirs, 1999 (1995).

Nightingale, Florence, *Notes on Nursing : what it is and what it is not*, London : Harrison, 1946 (1859).

Nuland, Sherwin B., "An Experience Both Physical and Spiritual," *Newsweek*, 19 May 2003, p. 62.

Nuland, Sherwin B., *The mysteries within: a surgeon reflects on medical myths*, New York: Simon & Schuster, 2000.

Odoul, Michel, *Dis-moi où tu as mal, je te dirai pourquoi*, Paris : Éditions France Loisirs, 2002.

Ornish, Dean, *Love and Survival, the Scientific Basis for the Healing Power of Intimacy*, New York : Harper Collins, 1998.

Oxenford, Rosalind, *Healing with reflexology, A concise guide to foot and hand massage for enhanced health and wellbeing*, London: Hermes House, 2003 (2002).

Pallardy, Pierre, *Et si ça venait du ventre?*, Paris : Robert Laffont, 2002.

Platon, *Œuvres complètes*, Volumes 1 and 2, translation by Léon Robin, Paris : Bibliothèque de la Pléiade, 1953 and 1955.

Quinn, Susan, *Human Trials, Scientists, Investors and Patients in the Quest for a Cure*, Cambridge (Massachusetts): Perseus Publishing, 2001.

Ricard, Matthieu, *Plaidoyer pour le bonheur*, Paris: Éditions France Loisirs, 2003.

Robert, Véronique, "Comment l'esprit peut guérir le corps," *Châtelaine*, September 2001, p. 36 – 44.

Roberto, Claude M., "My Garden," *The Gardener's Gate*, 2003, p. 5 – 7.

Rollot, Florence, *Le grand méchant stress*, Éditions de l'Homme, 2003.

Rosenberg, Charles E., *Florence Nightingale on Hospital Reform*, New York : Garland Publishing, 1989.

Rosenfeld, Isadore, *Guide to Alternative Medicine*, New York: Random House, 1996.

Roy, Monique, "L'Insouciance perdue," *Châtelaine*, May 2000, p.

49 – 52.

Saint-Arnaud, Yvon, *La guérison par le plaisir*, Ottawa: Novalis, 2002.

Servan-Schreiber, David, *Guérir le stress, l'anxiété et la dépression sans médicaments ni psychanalyse*, Paris : Éditions France Loisirs, 2003.

Siegel, Bernie S., *Peace, Love and Healing, Body Mind Communication and the Path to Self-Healing: An Exploration*, New York: Harper Collins, 2001 (1989).

Simpkins, C. Alexander and Simpkins, Annellen, *Self-hypnosis plain and simple*, Boston: Journey Editions, 2001.

Sophokles, *The Complete Plays*, translated by Carl R. Mueller and Anna Krajewska-Wieczorek, Hanover: Smith and Kraus, 2000.

Springen, Karen, "Helping the Littlest Patients," *Newsweek*, 19 May 2003, p. 54 – 61.

Stamatos, John M. with Jane O'Boyle, *Pain-buster, A Breakthrough 4-step program for ending chronic pain*, New York: Henry Holt and Company, 2001.

Stanton, Danielle, "Prière et guérison: un tissu de mensonges," *Actualité*, 15 September 2002, p. 57 – 62.

Stein, Joel, "Just say Om," *Time*, 3 August 2003, p. 37 – 46.

Stratton Hill, C., "The Negative Influence of Licensing and Disciplinary Boards and Drug Enforcement Agencies on Pain Treatment with Opioid Analgesics," *Journal of Pharmaceutical Care in Pain and Symptom Control*, Volume 1 (1), 1993, p. 43 – 62.

Sussman, Paul S., "No-Teacher No-Healer No-Doctor No-Therapist Bringing it All Back Home: One Private Practice in Heart-Centered Therapy," *Journal of Heart-Centered Therapy*, Volume 5, Number 1 Spring 2002, p. 98 – 131.

Sussman, Paul S. and Ferguson, H. B., "Elements of Early Avoidance Training and Relearning of Forgotten Operants," *Developmental Psychobiology*, Volume 13 (5), 1980, p. 545 – 562.

Taylor, Louise and Bryant, Betty, *Acupressure, Yoga and You*, Tokyo and New York: Japan Publications Inc., 1984.

Teasell, Robert W. and Merskey, Harold, "Chronic Pain Disability in the Workplace," *Pain Res Manage*, Volume 2, No 4, Winter 1997, p. 197 – 205.

The Merck Manual of Medical Information, Second Home Edition, Whitehouse Station, New Jersey: Merck & Co., Inc., 2003.

Tunks, Eldon, "Nonspecificity of Chronic Soft Tissue Pain Syndromes," *Pain Res Manage*, Volume 2, No 3, Autumn 1997, p.176 – 180.

Underwood, Anne, "An "Imaginary" Ailment that's all too real," *Newsweek*, 19 May 2003, p. 53.

Underwood, Nora, "The Placebo effect, when nothing really works," *Elm Street*, May 2003, p. 61 – 66.

Vicinus, Martha and Nergaard, Bea, *Ever Yours, Florence Nightingale, Selected letters*, Cambridge : Harvard University Press, 1990.

Washnis, George J. and Hricak, Richard Z., *Discovery of Magnetic Health, A Health Care Alternative*, Rockville: Nova Publishing Company, 1998 (1993).

Watt-Watson, Judith H., Clark, A. John, Finley, G. Allen, Watson, C. Peter N., "Canadian Pain Society Position Statement on Pain Relief," *Pain Res Manage*, Volume 4, No 2, Summer 1999, p. 75 – 78.

Wells, Chris and Nown, Graham, *The Pain Relief Handbook: Self-Help Methods for Managing Pain*, United Kingdom: Ebury Press, 1998.

Whichello Brown, Denise, *Réflexologie par les mains, une introduction pratique*, traduction d'Annie Chauveau, Laval: Les Publications Modus Vivendi, 2001.

Zolner, Theresa, "Workplace Bullying," *Seba Good News*, 2003, p. 8 – 17.

Note: Additional credit to Web sites is given within the book.